GW01418187

cancer with a small 'c'

cancer with a small 'c'

By

Elizabeth Caush

ISBN: 978-0-9930913-4-6

This book is published by Elizabeth Caush in conjunction with **WRITERSWORLD**, and is produced entirely in the UK. It is available to order from most bookshops in the United Kingdom, and is also globally available via UK based Internet book retailers.

Cover design by Jag Lall

Copy edited by Ian Large

WRITERSWORLD
2 Bear Close Flats, Bear Close, Woodstock
Oxfordshire, OX20 1JX, England
☎ 01993 812500
☎ +44 1993 812500

www.writersworld.co.uk

The text pages of this book are produced via an independent certification process that ensures the trees from which the paper is produced come from well managed sources that exclude the risk of using illegally logged timber while leaving options to use post-consumer recycled paper as well.

Some names and places have been changed to protect anonymity.

contents

For Edward

prologue

when did it all go wrong?

The dog looked up pathetically at me. His type of questioning look that I knew only too well meant that he was ready to go for the morning walk.

I felt tired. Bored of the simple routine of everyday life. I was always out of bed first in the morning. I made the tea. I walked the dog. I cleaned up the kitchen after everyone else, did the washing, ironing and generally kept the show on the road. Would anyone notice if I wasn't there anymore? Would anyone care? What wouldn't get done?

I clipped the lead onto Dougal's collar as his tail wagged enthusiastically in anticipation of exercise, fresh air and a change of environment. At least it wasn't raining. We took the usual route, my dog and I. We could have been alone in the world, each with our individual thoughts.

We could have gone a different way I suppose, but the familiarity of the path, side roads, crossings and general scenery propped me up with a sense of being grounded. Security. The opposite environment to the house I had just left.

We trudged along through the September breeze and every time the dog stopped to cock his leg I paused to invite another thought into my mind, encouraging it to develop into something bigger, more concrete. A plan.

As I urged the dog onwards with a quick pull on his lead, he looked knowingly up at me and we started on the homeward trail. If I didn't leave the house by a quarter to, I'd be late for work. I hated being late for anything. We still had to get indoors, wipe the pooch's paws, put his breakfast down, change his water – all this I did as if on autopilot. It was the regular routine. Unseen. Unacknowledged, except by the animal himself who would be the first to greet me home at the door the other end of the day.

I left the house with a 'see you later' shouted up the stairs, wondering how many other people would be doing exactly the same that morning in their own homes. Every morning.

chapter one

diagnosis and preparation

I once told my daughter that women are brave and very strong; this is what I needed to remind myself when I was first diagnosed with breast cancer. Those of us who have been through the experience of being advised that we are carrying a cluster of cancerous cells which need to be removed from our body will know exactly what I mean when I say that you never forget the time you were first told.

It's a bit like finding out that you are pregnant – your life will never be the same again. These are, obviously, totally opposite situations in terms of emotion and the physical side of the change. Confirmation of a pregnancy is usually positive and happy with an extra lump you don't mind carrying around for nine months, whilst the latter is nowhere near happy and the lump has to be got rid of as soon as possible. However, depending on circumstances, the latter could also apply to both situations.

At the time, I distanced myself from what was happening to my body. It affected only a tiny part of my body (I am a slightly built woman) and therefore it would simply be a little operation, after which I would be fine and return to work in a couple of weeks. I actually distanced myself from many things, a lot of which I really don't understand now as I reflect back on that time.

I drove my small, red Aygo along the tree-lined driveway that circled around the back of the old, red-bricked hospital and parked in the 'Visitors Only' car park. I was only a visitor and had no intention of returning after this appointment was over. It was a pleasant area, well attended shrubs and a small grassed roundabout in the middle of the car park accommodated several white Gerbera daisies standing to attention. I had read that the Georgian Grade II listed building, completed in 1762, was set in over sixty acres of land. There was something about its historic presence that gave off an air of authority. A safe place to be. Several expensive cars languished in the October sunlight, waiting for their owners' return. This could have been the car park of an expensive luxury hotel somewhere in the country. But it wasn't.

Never wanting to be late for anything, I had arrived early and remained seated in the car. Leaning my head back onto the headrest, closing my eyes and concentrating on my breathing, I waited for the allotted hour to come round. In for four, hold for four and out through the mouth for seven. That's what an article in one of those women's magazines at the hairdressers recommended and I didn't even think to question it. It always resulted in a calming effect so it must be right. My own thoughts and the reassurance of my sister convinced me that I was going to be fine, but there was always a sneaky doubt in my mind.

The afternoon sun dappled the vehicles through the trees as it made its lazy way through the clouds in an otherwise blue sky. Despite all the cars around me, I felt that there was no one else on the earth except me at that moment in time. Nobody came out to the vehicles and no new ones entered the car park. I was, at that point it felt, the only living being there. By myself.

The digits on the interior clock face rounded to 1500. It was always five minutes ahead of time, just to ensure that I was never late for appointments. Time to go. I hesitated for a moment, but then decided to take the bull by the horns and get this over and done with.

I stepped out of the car with my bag on my shoulder, slammed the door shut in a determined manner and pressed the remote button on my key fob to lock the doors. A reassuring clunk confirmed that the car was secure and would still be there waiting for me after the appointment. Head held high, I strutted in my high heels along the gravel towards the main entrance as I felt the warming autumn sun on my cheeks.

Eventually, I reached the heavy front door, which needed both hands and all my strength to open. 'Why aren't these doors fitted with automatic openings?' I thought, as I pushed the oak away from me. There are people less able than me who will have to battle their way in.

Once inside, two receptionists immediately looked up at me. I don't like it when more than one pair of eyes check me out. It's unsettling. To overcome this, I've learnt to put my shoulders back and offered them both a broad smile. Deep breath and state my name and appointment time – just wanting to get on with it, really.

"Date of birth," one of the women demanded.

"Twenty, six, fifty three," I replied proudly. Several people had told me that I don't look anywhere near my age and that I was far too young to have a daughter *that* age, and how did I manage to keep so young looking and on and on. It was great to have these compliments and I had now just started to believe them. I looked after myself. My mother brought me and my two sisters up to look after our skin and walk nicely. My older sister worked for one of the big cosmetic houses so there were always plenty of free samples available to use in the house I grew up in. How I missed my sister, especially at times like this. She would know how to handle it all. She'd gone through it all herself and was so brave. But I was alone now and I wanted to do this on my own.

It's worth mentioning here that our eldest sister had breast cancer, and then SEVENTEEN years later was diagnosed with liver cancer. She was 'given' eighteen months but died three years on from that date. Positive attitude.

The receptionist looked at me again in confusion and her colleague also looked up. Yes, dear, I am fifty four, I thought to myself. It's years of Clarins, early nights and a vegetarian diet. And, of course, Mother's wisdom.

"Please confirm your address," the woman continued in a dour tone. I always give people the benefit of the doubt when they seemed to be miserable and the thought briefly swept through my mind that perhaps this woman didn't have a happy home life. Her po-faced expression gave away her inside feelings only too well. Deidre, her badge announced. Deidre Dolldrums. Erase that thought, it's unkind, I told myself.

Here we go, I thought.

"Well, I used to live in Sutton Road but I'm staying with my sister at the moment, so my actual address now is Nash Drive, although I will be moving again soon." I immediately realised this was too much information for Deidre to compute.

"So where should we send correspondence to?" Po-face

8

continued her expressionless tirade of questions.

I know it's confusing, but keep up, Deidre Dear, I thought but said, "Nash Drive, please. Number twenty one," accompanied by another wide, red-lipped smile flashing my white, even teeth. I looked after those too!

"Take a seat through there," Deidre commanded, indicating an archway with her left hand while her gaze dropped back down to the paperwork on her desk.

"Thank you," I replied in the most pleasant voice I could muster.

I walked through the narrow archway, which opened into a small, dingy and isolated waiting room. A direct opposite of the exterior garden area, this room was unkempt, unloved. As I sat down on one of the plastic covered seats I considered how many other people had sat in the same place. How many poor, unsuspecting patients had died after sitting in this chair. Depressing. Someone had tried to cheer up the area by pinning posters to the wall and an attempt had been made with a few artificial flowers in a plastic vase, but their aged expression suggested that this had happened a long time ago. Staff shortage, I thought, or cut backs.

"Elizabeth Couch?" A bright-eyed, smiling woman with cropped red hair summoned me.

"Yes, that's me." I picked up my bag, stood and followed the crop of red hair out of the room, quietly excusing her mispronunciation of my surname. It was often a problem. Should have married someone called 'Smith'. I remember thinking that I had been called in very quickly and that maybe it wouldn't take so long after all. Home for a cup of tea soon. Well, temporary home but definitely a cup of tea.

"I just need to weigh you." The red head's white tunic top instilled a degree of confidence in me as I stood on the ancient platform of the scales. It was clear that the old-fashioned piece of equipment had started off life dark green, but over many years the paint had worn away in the same place where thousands of women had stood and held onto the horizontal bar to steady themselves, just as I did. Over the years, women had stood here just before they were told the best news ever, or the worst. This was just the beginning, if it wasn't positive news. But I remained convinced that I was ok. It was all going to be alright.

"Sixty two kay," was the verdict, and noticing my attempt at working out my weight in 'old money' as some called it, red head came to my rescue and pointed to the conversion chart in front of me.

"Oh, thanks." I felt stupid for not having noticed this before and even worse as I squinted to find the right box. I knew I ought to have my spectacles with me at all times but somehow they always seemed to be in the wrong place. Like now, in my handbag on the floor, out of reach. I'd calculate it on my phone later but had a feeling that I would have to keep my diet in check from now on. This sounded like a danger of brushing too close to the edge of ten stone. That was more than I wanted for my height.

I stepped off the scales and was directed to take another seat around the corner. Around the corner there was a long line of people sitting on chairs against the wall, as if waiting for the firing squad to arrive, ready for their individual verdict. Most were accompanied by a friend, partner, husband, mother or had some sort of empathic supporter with them. I wanted to do this on my own. I didn't need anyone. I needed to show other people that I was strong. The saying that I'd told my daughter many times came to mind once again. Women are brave and very strong. Now I had to be both. On my own.

I placed myself on the only vacant chair, between a young looking woman who was with her husband and another older woman who looked very scared. I smiled at the latter who blinked back a resigned smile as if the inevitable was in sight.

The yellowing framed print of Constable's *Hay Wain* hanging on the wall did nothing to improve the area; nor did the posters advocating early detection of breast cancer and how it could save lives if found early enough. There was a self-help group advertising relaxation courses and regular meetings for support. No, I thought, I won't be needing this, and turned to my neighbour in an attempt to strike up conversation.

"Have you been waiting long?" I gently asked the scared

looking woman.

"About twenty minutes," the woman replied, consulting a tiny gold watch wrapped round her chubby wrist.

"Oh, not too bad then." I thought that this was going to be like pulling teeth.

"No, they're usually quite good here."

"Is... is this not your first time, then?" I asked gingerly.

"No. No," the woman replied, "it came back. Had the op and all was fine, then back it came. Ravished me."

I was unsure what to say at this point, so put on my empathic expression reserved for those who had suffered bereavement. And it is a kind of bereavement to lose a part of one's body, however small, and from an intimate place at that.

"Mind you," the older woman continued, "they're very good. Very good here, you know."

I smiled in gratitude for the consolation but was sure that it wouldn't come to that in my case. This was just a routine check. To check all was well, not to find out that all was *not* well.

"Mrs Smith." The cropped red hair appeared from the next room. "This way, dear."

Mrs Smith pushed down on the arms of the chair to haul her considerable weight up to a standing position and followed the nurse, reconciled to another operation looming on the horizon.

Being ill or needing an operation wasn't an option for me. I would carry on my life regardless of what my body told me. I can cope. It would be fine. Anyway, I ran the department at work and no one else would be able to do that. An operation would demand far too much time to be taken away from the office and I needed the money. Well, I would need the money now I'd left my husband. I was going to have to be able to support myself without him. The job was a necessity, not a luxury any more.

It was all very new, this being on my own business. I continued to think about what the future could hold. The many possibilities. I'd left him in circumstances that he seemed to understand, but not support. My feelings for him were odd now, not like they used to be thirty or so years ago.

"But people change," a friend had told me.

"You're married for life," my sister reminded me, but still offered to let me stay at their house while I went through whatever this consultation was going to reveal.

"I wish my parents had split rather than stay together and be really miserable until my dad died and then mum became an alcoholic," another friend confided.

Everyone had a different story depending on their circumstances. But everyone was individual and had a right to a life that was... that was what? Tolerable? Enjoyable? I wasn't sure any more. "You never know what goes on behind closed doors," I had been told. You never do, unless you're on the inside.

My husband was everything I wanted in a man, or so I thought. He was brave and ambitious, courageous and good looking. Other women looked at him in the street. Other women told me how lucky I was. And I knew it. However, there was always a 'but'. Nothing's perfect. Not in this life, anyway. The possessiveness and claustrophobia had become too much and I had to break away. Be myself, find myself... I didn't really know what that meant any more.

Now I was my own person. I would make my own decisions from now on and everything would be fine. It was strange at first but I was on the verge of moving into my own flat, and once there I knew I would feel better about things. Clearer. Time to call my own. Time to think about life and myself. It sounded selfish, but although I wanted to give out to others and had done so for a long time, I was becoming drained of energy to cope with everything else going on at home.

Time passed slowly as I sat there in the gloom, waiting for my name to be called. The couple seated the other side of Mrs Smith had gone into the consultant's room for their turn; surely I was going to be next. I leafed through the dog-eared pages of one of the well read magazines on the small table squeezed in between the chairs. The celebrities smiled their Botox out from the pages, while the journalists slated them, disclosed something private they would prefer to keep secret or praised their outfits – depending on who was paying them. I put the magazine back and swapped it for a more tasteful *House and Garden*, which, I knew, would make more pleasant reading. The azalea yellows promised fragrant yellow blooms late in the spring. I wondered how many of the women here today would still be around to see the next season. My mind meandered through the possibilities of having my own house, my own garden and planting azaleas in moist acidic soil as recommended in the magazine.

I was startled back into the waiting area by the now familiar chirpy voice of the redhead. "Mrs Court?" The rhetorical question required no reply as I was the only one left in the waiting area.

"Must be me!" I tried to sound cheerful but the long wait had dampened my mood and I was no longer sure if this appointment was going to be as I had hoped. However, I pulled myself quickly out of the malaise, stood up and dropped the *House and Garden* back onto the table with the rest of the hopeless pile of magazines.

"This way, Dr Palmer is in here for you."

I was led into another room, much bigger and lighter than either of the previous areas and there were more people in here. Important looking people. One of the breast care nurses, a couple of men in white coats who looked like doctors and a smaller man in a suit. I was asked to take a seat and immediately the suited man wheeled his office chair from behind a large desk to remove the barrier between us. I liked him immediately and it became obvious that everyone else in the room was only there because of me. This made me feel important, but I didn't understand why. It couldn't be good.

His kind eyes looked straight into mine. An expensive gold watch on his wrist and a small yellow handkerchief popping out from the top of his breast pocket confirmed his obvious wealth. My thoughts briefly considered how huge his monthly salary would be and that he probably lived a luxurious lifestyle to match. No wedding ring, though. Swiftly I returned to the present where he was smiling at me.

"Mrs Court." His tanned face and greying hair at the temples addressed me in a slightly sombre tone. Professional. Good.

I wanted to say, "Please, call me Elizabeth," but quickly realised this would be most inappropriate, so I just smiled at him in acceptance of another mispronunciation of my surname and raised my questioning eyebrows. The moment seemed to last longer than it should have. This was disconcerting. So I drew in a deep breath, sat upright with my shoulders back and prepared for the assault. I suddenly knew, *just knew* that this wasn't good. But it wasn't right, either.

oOoOoOoOo

I need to say at this point that we are all different and so are our experiences. During the research for this book I have met some marvellous people, all with a different story, and the majority were fighters when they needed to be – and positive in attitude years later when I asked them to reflect on their experiences. Some were told and found themselves in hospital very quickly; for others it took longer due to holidays booked and a feeling of being in control of *something* – that was one of my feelings, being out of control of what was happening.

The oncologist's very words to me were, "I'm afraid it's a malignant tumour." Now I considered myself an intelligent woman at that time in my fifties, but I didn't understand what he meant. What was a 'tumour'? What did 'malignant' mean – was that the good sort or not? I just couldn't think straight. The blood rushed to my head and I must have gone very red. I took a deep breath and one of the breast care nurses came over to me and held my hand. This had to mean it was bad.

"I can't have an operation this month," I stammered, grasping at something that I could be in control of, if only the timing of what was going to happen. My thoughts dashed through what was going on at work, at home, my children, the dog. Everything became very muddled.

"Did you come here today with someone?" A kindly, bedside manner accompanied this question from the nurse.

"No... no, I'm on my own. But I'll be ok. It's ok." It was probably the self-reassurance that I was practising. That would be repeated many times in the future.

As I eventually walked out to the car park, returning to my car, it felt like I was someone else. Sort of walking on air, not really with it, and by putting one foot in front of the other wondered how I had transported myself to the vehicle. Even my car looked different. Others may sense some resonance with these feelings I was going through. A natural reaction to shock. It is also natural to initially think that they've got it wrong, mixed up my X-rays with someone else's or just to simply not believe them.

Another lady told me that she had also received her news on her own and had walked home to her husband, but didn't know how she got there.

One of the questions on the sheet I widely distributed to find out about other people's experiences when they were first diagnosed with breast cancer asked, "Can you describe your feeling at the time?" Various different responses came back, but a common theme was overwhelmingly similar, using words such as: devastated, shocked, disbelief, upset. It will have been something that none of us had been through before when we hear this for the first time. Needless to say, it is bound to be distressing to an enormous degree but the general feeling of your head belonging to someone else and detached from your body is, I was told, quite a normal reaction. I have likened it to a bad car crash, when at first you are driving along happily and the entire surrounding environment is familiar, everything is where it should be and subconsciously you feel safe. Then, suddenly and unexpectedly, the environment changes to such an extent that you don't know where you are any more. The steering wheel and dashboard are close to your face and eyes, you're upside down, possessions have fallen out of their holds and there is chaos everywhere. Nothing is in its right place.

A similar feeling may be experienced by the person who has received the news that they have breast cancer. Nothing about it seems right. Everything is upside down. Suddenly faced with a chaos that needs immediate attention. Inevitably, feeling it has to be sorted quickly.

I read in a magazine that today, one hundred and thirty women will be diagnosed with breast cancer in the UK. That's over a hundred different reactions, different responses and behaviours. Over a hundred families who will be affected. Some people have more supportive families and friends than others; some are surrounded by loving, caring and well-meaning people, which is great if that's what's needed at the time. I wanted to be left alone, and I know that isn't everyone's feeling – indeed, I will readily acknowledge that it was probably me who was the odd one out. And I know that I hurt many people with my selfish response to some of their offers. Perhaps I can take this opportunity to once again express my sorrow on this point. There was a lot of 'making up' I had to do once I had come through and out the other end of my dark tunnel.

During the time that led up to my hospital admission I became more aware of this little extra lump I was carrying around with me in my breast. It was there when I woke up in the mornings, when I went to bed at night and sometimes even in my dreams. It doesn't go away. I discussed with my breast care nurse the possibility of just leaving it alone; maybe it would become less important. She kindly dissuaded me from this line of thought and, as she described what could happen, it left me in no doubt that I had to have it removed.

Apparently, it continues to grow and can even force its way outside the skin, developing a nasty smell because an open tumour can bleed, ooze fluid and become infected. Horrible to think of, but surely not an option when considering a mastectomy or lumpectomy. These operations are something you will, undoubtedly, get through somehow, whereas if you just leave it and hope for the best you have no idea what is round the corner.

According to one website, 'most breast lumps are benign' (not a threat to life or long-term health, especially by being non-cancerous). Benign breast tumours are abnormal growths, but they do not spread outside of the breast. So if this is the conclusion of your diagnosis, great, you won't have to go through anything major at the moment and maybe never. However, this book is an attempt to reassure and comfort those who have had a diagnosis like mine – it *is* breast cancer.

A shock, yes, but take each day as it arrives and work your way through what is being thrown at you with whatever help you need. Offers of help and support will be there and you need to accept them and not be too proud to be helped. The saying 'what goes around, comes around' has some validity here. There will be someone else in a similar situation to where you are now that you can help in the future, or may have already helped in the past. Now it is your turn to be accepting of what lies ahead. It is scary, but you can manage it and get through it.

As I prepared for my admission into hospital, I remember what seems now to be the stupidest things I wanted to sort out beforehand. Nothing to do with remaking my will or sorting out the children or the things that would remain outstanding while I was absent, but it was work. Who would do what needed to be done while I was away? I worked late into the evenings and tried to make everything as clear as I could for others to pick up. It was as if I thought I was indispensable, which, of course, I was not. No one is. Not even if you think your business, office, school, family or whatever depends entirely on you – you must face up to the fact that when you are not around, someone else will do the essentials. Even if it is the minimum and not how you would do it, it will – or will not – get done. Right now there is nothing else you can do about it, so sit back and enjoy the rest!

I have a suspicion that my stress levels whilst working at the college were (at the time of my diagnosis) at an all-time high. My husband tried to tell me that, but when you're in the thick of it and are enthusiastic about your work, it's difficult to hear what others are saying to you. I worked late, came home and did more work and collapsed into bed at an unearthly hour, wondering why I was so tired but couldn't sleep. Our marriage was being stretched to its limits and beyond. My mind was not functioning rationally and I did the only thing I thought I could do and that was to walk away from everything.

chapter two

preparation – she's leaving home

No one's marriage is perfect. If they tell you it is, they're lying! Those who survive this institution and make it last have to draw on reserves of tolerance, patience and grace. At this point in my life all of the above ran out. I had come to the end of everything. I just wanted out.

My husband was, to my eyes and ears, being very critical of the type and amount of food I was eating. Ok, I have a sweet tooth and I love chocolate but I can make my own decisions. It's my body. He did not concur. Feeling like an alcoholic with chocolate replacing the booze, I would hide it in cupboards, bags, anywhere I thought he wouldn't find it. He probably did find some. Not only that but other unhelpful and, quite honestly, downright abusive comments he made directly to me were beginning to ruffle my feathers and I wondered why I ever decided to marry him in the first place. This was my state of mind at the time.

It's the kids. Women often stay in a marriage for the kids, with no thought of putting themselves first. In my case, I always tried to put others first. Joy. But now things had gone too far. I was working all hours, stressing out about my job, kids, money and never having enough time for anything I wanted to do.

"You must calm down," I was told from a variety of others. No one is indispensable. I knew the words but who exactly is going to cover my shift on the rotas at church, check that the course is set up properly at work, type my husband's letters and do his accounts, walk the dog and take him to the vet? Who? When? Some of these things carried deadlines, which if not reached would cause catastrophic effects. Not on a worldwide basis and probably no one would die, but it would cause distress to others. For instance, I can't see the tax man waiting for his money just because I hadn't got my husband's business figures to our accountant on time. A class full of adult learners waiting for a tutor who hasn't turned up could affect their perception of education – worse when it was an exam and the papers weren't there. Manic.

So a decision was made. Correction: I made a decision. I packed a few clothes and things I thought I would need and left. Left my husband, my children, my dog and my church. Initially, my sister said to move in with her and her husband. They had no children, just two black cats and a big house. It made sense to go there for a while, so that's what I did. I continued to go to work, eat, sleep, and life kept going on around me. Me in my cosmoses. Only it wasn't ordered, my mind was muddled and had to keep going on a type of automatic pilot, convincing myself that my children (now 20 and 25 – young adults) didn't need me and nor did anyone else. Everything and everyone survived.

Well, nearly everything, maybe the odd potted plant wilted. The dog wasn't walked nearly enough and his coat needed a good brush by the time I saw him again. Our daughter moved to London – proof that I wasn't the lovely mother she desperately wanted to be near every day. Our son turned to drugs – or rather *re*turned – he'd been smoking cannabis for years and I thought he'd stopped but maybe he never did and possibly never would. Other people had to step in and fill my slots on the church rotas. I shouldn't have taken on so much. My husband had to pay someone to come in and type his letters. Only she couldn't do the accounts like I did and her keyboard skills and grammar were rubbish. What a mess.

But what did I care? I wasn't going back so they could all just get on with it. Strangely enough, I didn't crave chocolate and yet I was in a position where I could eat anything I wanted. I lost a bit of weight and had a major operation looming. Just anxiety...

In the early 1600s John Donne wrote, "No man is an island," and actually, this is quite true. However, there are times when some of us want to be just that. No phone calls, texts or emails, please. Just leave me alone. Donne pointed out that we are inextricably linked to other people, and as part of mankind we all share in suffering. Empathy. Some people can do it but others don't seem to be gifted in the same way. It is the latter that I mainly wanted rid of. Stay away with your trite phrases and sympathetic looks enquiring if I was 'alright' and reassuring me that I was 'missed'. I didn't care. Pray for me all you like if it makes you feel better. The letters and cards and flowers I received were overwhelming. Yes, all from people who wanted to help me but not understanding that I didn't want them bothering me. Maybe they felt better.

It's really difficult to know how much to tell people that you care for them. One of the most honest letters I received at the time simply stated, 'I don't know what to say.' Honesty. You just need to be honest, rather than trot out the phrases that you may have heard others say. Donne was right; we all feel the need to connect with each other in some way. How many of us can walk past on the other side when we see someone suffering – especially if we know of someone (or even ourselves) who have suffered something similar? Then the tales and the stories begin, some of which may be encouraging, but others describe how dreadful things are or could be, or worse.

How selfish a time that was; I can see it now as I reflect on the texts I deleted, the messages I never replied to, the cards carrying good wishes I simply put in the bin. As a child in Sunday school I remember being taught that 'JOY' stood for Jesus first, Others next and Yourself last. Now, as an adult, I had not only reversed those letters but completely deleted the first two. It was all about me, the egocentric self.

In my defence, looking back at that time from where I am now, ten years later, I simply don't recognise myself. It's a strange thing, illness, disability, disease. They all play with your mind. The neural pathways receive messages that are forwarded on in an often bizarre and strange manner. A manner that we just don't recognise as normal. Whatever normal is. We all have our own 'normals', just as we all have our own pain thresholds and respond differently to shock, whether it's shocking news or a physical trauma.

The operation date loomed ever closer and I felt a little similar to the time just before I went into labour with our first baby. The thought that my life would never be the same again. And it wouldn't. Through time, my self-description moved from 'I have cancer' to 'I've had cancer'. In between I suppose I was 'living with cancer', and living I was – not from my sick bed, but carrying on as normally as possible. Yes, I was tired but this was also due to work overload and my mind exploring different possibilities regarding the outcome after the operation, after the divorce. The next few months, years even, grasped at my unknown.

All the leaflets and information I was given from the hospital were very reassuring and made an attempt at letting me know how I was going to feel and what was going to happen and all the rest of it. No one, not even the experts can tell you how you are going to feel. It was a journey into an unfamiliar experience and I was going to be brave and do this on my own. I am a woman. I am brave and very strong. That was my mantra at the time. Tell yourself a positive fact enough times over and you will come to believe it. The opposite is also true – keep telling yourself that you can't do something and you won't. We can do anything. It just has to be believed. Well, maybe a bit more than that, but this was my thinking at the time.

One piece of advice from the NHS literature was not to go out and buy new nighties prior to an operation. During this phase, when I was questioning everything and disputing most facts, I went out and bought the most beautiful negligee set. Two new nighties and a lovely, light, cream, floating dressing gown. I knew that hospitals were hot places so I wanted to be cool, comfortable and stylish. And yes, I would bring in some lipstick and a little bit of blusher. Pack that mascara, too. I've never worn a lot of make-up, but I intended to look 'ok' and ready to receive visitors, if any were to dare come into my vicinity. I had to tell the doctors, friends, visitors, the whole world, that I was doing alright. That I had survived.

The preparation for an operation such as this involves a forest of paper. Forms to give consent, next of kin, blood pressure – oh dear, the blood pressure. It was up and they weren't prepared to operate on someone with such a high score. There followed a period of abstinence from tea (tannin), coffee (caffeine) and chocolate (sugar) accompanied by the strongest withdrawal headaches I have ever experienced. Perhaps I did overindulge in these daily luxuries but I didn't realise just how much.

The operation actually takes very little time compared with others on a grander scale. Consequently, although I applaud the surgeons and all medical and nursing staff, I will not devote a whole chapter to this part of the story.

The morning arrived when I was not allowed any breakfast. Fasting. I reminded myself to fast more often, it really felt quite good – once you get past the 'I'm hungry' stage. It's cleansing and seemed to clear my mind.

My sister drove me to the hospital along with my little case of things I thought I may need. Again, we're all different in our needs so the contents of my case may not be typical, but I gave some things more priority. I knew I would write, so a huge pad of writing paper and a few pens were essential. I also took what was quite possibly an overdose of pants, and there's another story.

I went into one of the cheap shops to buy some knickers, thinking that I could just throw them away if they didn't survive my hospital stay. Not sure of my thought process there, but served by a young man at the cash desk I felt a need to explain to him why I was buying so many pairs of pants.

"I'm going into hospital, you know. Big operation." I smiled and looked him straight in the eyes. He smiled. "Actually I have breast cancer and I don't know how long I'm going to be in for." This was too much information and the young cashier was clearly placed out of his comfort zone so he just smiled and nodded again. Looking back on that exchange, I can imagine him in the pub that night with his mates recalling the tale of an old biddy who wanted to spill the beans about her op. At the time, I had absolutely no thought for others, whoever they were. My operation, the cancer, was digging in and making me feel sorry for myself, yet simultaneously making me want to tell the whole world that it was ok and I would cope with this.

I also packed some CDs, a great asset not only for me but my companion patients. Someone lent me a portable CD player and some ear phones. Good move. Mobile phone, of course, and charger. Bank card and a bit of money – why? If my stay didn't go according to plan, I would escape, drawing out all the money I had and just disappear. Clearly, this was not a well thought through plan, but it was there in my mind.

Then I decided to consult the list I had been given: 'What to pack for your stay in hospital.' This included:

- a nightdress or pyjamas
- day clothes
- reading glasses
- clean underwear
- dressing gown and slippers
- small hand towel
- toiletries – soap, toothbrush, toothpaste, shampoo, deodorant
- sanitary towels or tampons
- razor and shaving materials
- comb or hairbrush
- book or magazines
- small amount of money
- medication you normally take, and a list of the doses for each medicine
- notebook and pen
- healthy snacks
- address book and important phone numbers, including your GP's contact details

No lipstick then! But there you are, we all pack what we want to because we're all different.

chapter three

admission and discharge

My sister drove me to the hospital and we arrived in plenty of time, even though it was extremely early in the morning. I was asked some questions by various medical staff and directed to sign a form. We were shown to another room and I was asked my full name and date of birth. This seemed to be repeated several times: questions, forms, signatures. At last we were shown to the bed that was allocated to me. My sister and I sat side by side on the edge of the bed in silent resignation.

"Now, who's the patient?" The cheery, nursey voice belonged to a plump lady in a blue uniform. There was a chart on the wall that clearly stated what colour uniform signified the grade of nurse. I hadn't read it, so I didn't know. Did it matter, anyway? This new person was going to be part of my journey and when it was all over, I would probably never see her again.

My sister laughed nervously, "Not me!" She pointed at me and leapt off the bed. Neither of us knew at that time what was in store for either of us. How can anyone know what's just around the corner? She was to have to undergo the same operation more than once in the future but we didn't have any idea at that time. We have to take life as it comes and deal with it as best we can. I try to always think of something positive or amusing to get me through tough times.

"Must be me, then." I tried to sound happy and put the whole event into some sort of perspective.

There was another round of name, date of birth collection and all that, a couple more signatures and then the gown was presented to me, accompanied by a "Just pop that on, opening down the back," from my nurse caretaker. How many times must she have said that in her life?

I did as I was told, my sister putting the clothes I took off dutifully into a bag I'd brought with me so that they could go straight in the wash at home. We were told prior to admission not to bring too much as the bedside lockers were small. At this point I panicked that two nighties weren't going to be enough, but my sister assured me that she would be in every day and could just take them home to wash one day and bring them back the next. That was ok then.

The nurse then re-appeared. They seem to have a practised skill at whipping the curtains back round the steel rail, a bit like ripping off a plaster so that it doesn't hurt so much. I felt very exposed in my back opening gown, although I had made sure that the opening was overlapping so nothing, in fact, was exposed.

"Ok, then, all ready?" I was asked.

"Well, yes, I suppose." What was I meant to reply to a question like this? Can't wait, let the party begin?

"Ah," the nurse said, with a look of concern veiling her face, "that'll have to come off."

Nail polish on my toes. But I always wore nail polish on my toes and sometimes even my fingers! This was not allowed in the hospital and most definitely not in theatre. The nurse bustled back with a small bottle and some cotton wool. I obeyed and removed the polish. Not that I had any other option, especially in an open backed gown!

My sister and I were discussing the necessity of removing nail polish before an operation when Nurse Efficient bustled round the corner and explained that, "Nail varnish can interfere with the monitors used to measure the oxygen in your blood during the operation. Sometimes the toes can be the area used to monitor oxygenation. It helps if a patient has no nail varnish on. Then, in theatre, you can be kept as safe as possible during the procedure." So then we knew. I have since been told that although there are now more sophisticated ways of measuring if you're alright during an operation, the finger nails are the first to show if your body is short of oxygen. I guess, as the 'procedure' is taking place at the top end of the body, maybe the toe nails give the same information.

So there we sat, my sister and I, on the edge of the hospital bed. I'm not sure who was the most anxious, because although the patient who goes through the operation is the one who receives the most attention, to be a bystander is also difficult. I know this because I have since been in my sister's place. The *Breast Cancer and You* booklet will tell you that 'Sometimes husbands and partners have difficulty dealing with what is happening too. They may become distant or cope by being very matter of fact.' Well my husband was out of the picture, so at least I wasn't putting him through the worry of all this. Of course, I had no way of knowing what he was going through and it probably made it harder that he didn't know my predicament. His line of communication was through my sister and she only told him what I allowed her to pass on.

I was second on the list that day. However, there was a flurry of activity when it was discovered that the person first on the list either hadn't turned up or had changed their mind. Not that one can change one's mind at this late stage, but something unexpected had happened and I was immediately promoted to the first on the list for the day. Very quickly I was ushered into the next room with a hasty 'goodbye' to my sister and reply from her, "We'll be praying for you." I didn't mind, I just wanted to get this out of the way, over and done with, so to be 'going down' so soon meant a lot less waiting time and I would be back up on the ward in time for the coffee break! No problem.

It was a surprise to me that I had to walk to the next station carrying two pillows and some forms. You go nowhere without forms prior to an op! As I was fit and able to walk, then I suppose that saved another person from having to wheel me in a chair – and two people if I was on a gurney.

After that I was asked if I'd like to get onto a trolley bed where I was made comfortable with my two pillows and one of those honeycomb blankets that all hospitals seem to have. They are, actually, a good blanket – light, breathable and warm enough. From here on I was, literally, in someone else's hands. In fact, in several other people's hands.

Now, can anyone tell me why it is that anaesthetists are always so good looking? Even in their scrubs, the ones I have seen all reach the 'highly attractive' mark on my scale. This day was no different. He chatted away to me and I told him in very enthusiastic terms how I loved my job and what I did and how busy I'd been lately and... and... as my words slurred me into a deep sleep, that was it.

I find sleeping and the effects of anaesthetics very interesting. Where do we go? What exactly happens to our minds while we drift onto another plane? Apparently scientists aren't exactly sure how they work, but work they do. A mixture of nitrous oxide and derivatives of ether such as isoflurane, sevoflurane and desflurane are precisely mixed together so that just the right amount is administered to get us all the way through the operation and no longer.

Needless to say, I cannot recount my experience on the operating table; all I can remember is that it seemed to be all over in a few seconds. Obviously, it took longer than that.

When I woke up, or rather tried to open my eyes, I heard someone saying, "Here she is, Sleeping Beauty." A blurred outline of someone in a green coat was moving gently around me, while in the background I could hear a conversation but couldn't make out the words. I gave in to my heavy eyelids and allowed them to close, blocking out where I was and what had happened. I felt the least like any kind of sleeping beauty, but it was a fun thing for him to say.

It was a strange situation when I was in the recovery room, on a trolley and yet not fully there. Not fully conscious. I could hear and see and smell and almost taste something, something unfamiliar and I was so, so tired. And thirsty. I desperately wanted a drink. Someone kept saying that they were getting me some water, but it felt like an extended period before it actually arrived. Then I could only have sips.

If you have ever been wheeled along hospital corridors on a trolley, you may relate to the feeling of being pushed along with your vision on the ceiling, bright lights rushing along above you and sounds coming from unknown places, all going to an unknown destination as the nursing staff help, transport and talk in kindly tones.

So that was it.

I know now that if your bed is nearest to the nursing station, it's because they're keeping an eye on you. Or something has gone wrong. The latter didn't occur to me and I began to feel quite comfortable knowing that the correct medical help was nearby.

I wanted to sit up but felt frightened to move. I wanted a cup of tea but felt that I had to wait. I wasn't totally sure where I was and certainly had no idea of which part of the Georgian Grade II listed building made up my surroundings.

As more patients were returned from the operating theatre and the day wore on, I was moved to another position on the ward. Everything must be ok, then, I thought, as my bed (with me still in it) was wheeled to a location further away from the nurses' station.

Now, I always find it hard to sit still, let alone lie in bed and do nothing. However, over the next couple of days I found that I didn't have the energy to stay awake long enough to do anything significant. Reading a book found me nodding off before I reached the end of the chapter. Journaling my experience similarly sent me back to sleep before I completed a sentence. There was nothing for it but to give in and rest. At times, you just have to 'go with it' and that means taking enforced rest when your body directs, even when you don't want to.

I didn't want to look at the site of my operation. All the nurses on the ward were kind and I discovered later that some of them had also been through the same operation. One particular nurse came to my bed and pulled the curtains round – I knew something was going to happen that wasn't for public display.

"Have you looked at your wound?" she asked, gently.

"No. No, I don't want to," I replied, fearful that she would make me.

"That's ok, just let me know when you're ready and we can do it together when I change the dressing."

How kind. How nice of her not to push me into doing something I absolutely didn't feel up to at that time. Clearly, I would have to look and face up to what had been done to my body, but not now. Even a small piece of control over that helped me to feel stronger, and the very next day I was able to let her know that I was ready.

We can't know exactly what to expect the site or sight of a

wound to look like and if, like me, you are at all squeamish then you won't have been used to looking at blood, guts, cuts and grazes or worse. Of course, there will be others who like to see what sort of suture the surgeon had used and whether it was neat and so on. We're not all the same. The nurses, fortunately for me, fell into the latter camp and were all in agreement that 'my' surgeon had performed a very precise cut and a tidy sewing up. Even their words made me want to faint.

Once again, I was ready to glance – only glance – at my post-op body and, you know, it wasn't that bad. Apparently my lymph glands needed to drain of all fluid. This involved two narrow tubes that were inserted somewhere in the region of my armpit and trailed down to outside the first beautiful nightie. Those of us with the 'drains' were each issued with a lovely, handmade, cotton bag with a shoulder strap. Mine had a blue, floral pattern adorning it. What a considerate act – someone had thought of this time (or maybe even gone through it themselves) and made an otherwise hideous and unsightly piece of apparatus into almost a thing of beauty. At least its carrier was a thing of beauty. The bag, obviously, had to come everywhere with me. It became a temporary companion! Once the drains had stopped draining, then they would be taken out. The bag was emptied once a day and a note made of how much of the fluid had actually drained away.

The woman in the bed next to me had a kind face and so I decided to strike up a conversation. I wish I could remember her name now, but although we kept in touch for a while after discharge, inevitably we lost contact as our lives moved on. Friends come into our lives for a reason, a season or a lifetime, so the poem goes. In hospital – and come to that, on holiday or in work – I don't usually make friends. Maybe my life is too compartmentalised, but I prefer it that way. For me, friends are friends and work is work – keep them separate. So I had no intention of making a lifetime friend of this person who happened to be in the next bed to me, but I thought it may make our time in the hospital a little more bearable if we shared stories and carried out the hospital issued page of exercises together.

My first instinct was correct, she was a kind soul. We must have been about the same age; she may have been a few years younger than me, but we got along with small talk and chit chat about life, children, pets and that sort of thing.

We both had our floral shoulder bags enclosing the drains and each day as our liquid egress was measured, we compared notes. As we were encouraged to get out of bed, we would gather together a couple of other women and go on an adventure to the shop which was a few minutes' walk within the hospital site. However, there was a whiteboard mounted on the wall just inside the ward on which we were instructed to write our names, the time and where we were going. I understand that we had to account for our comings and goings but I seemed to revert to my mischievous younger self at this point. I would write the correct time on the board and the names of the patients who were with me, but under 'Destination' I invariably wrote 'Harrods', 'Paris' and other similar places. The staff knew my jokes and I think were pleased with how I rallied others round to move and go outside. After all, we only had our dressing gowns in which to walk across the open courtyard! So we couldn't go far, but it gave us a tiny fraction of independence. Control. Even that was tiring and we would all return half an hour later, lay on our beds and inevitably fall asleep for a couple of hours. Never underestimate how much an operation, or maybe it's the anaesthetic, takes out of you. I have never felt so tired in my life and I don't think I ever will again.

When I discovered that there was an area at the end of the ward that was to be used for patients who wanted to sit quietly or read (and more importantly it contained a working CD player), I had an idea. We were all supposed to do the pages of certain exercises daily, but I never saw many others carrying out their daily workout. So I visited everyone in bed and asked them if they would be interested in a gentle exercise get together at the end of the ward. Eleven o'clock, then we wouldn't miss the coffee round. I played one of my CDs, nothing too jazzy but it was upbeat enough to do our exercises. And most of my fellow bed patients joined in. At the end of the exercise session we collapsed in the armchairs and I remember that I played a Katherine Jenkins CD as we sat in companionable silence, some with their eyes closed. One older woman thanked me for adding a little light to her day. That's all I needed to hear – it became a daily routine. Some patients needed more encouragement than others, but generally our little session was welcomed. It also meant that people had to get out of bed, interact with others and move, instead of just lying in or on a bed waiting for the day they could go home.

The visitors I received were interesting. I always applied a bit of lipstick just before visiting time and did something with my hair so that they would observe a woman who had gone through surgery and was now making a full, rapid and complete recovery. I didn't want anyone to worry or fuss, but I did enjoy the attention the visits brought. Flowers were not usually accepted in the hospital but my work colleagues sent the biggest bunch you can image. Beautifully wrapped and with the obligatory box of chocolates when the buyer pays an extra five pounds, I felt truly loved and missed. They knew me well. Apart from more chocolates, sweets and magazines I also received some very practical gifts. Wet wipes to freshen up when I didn't feel like leaving my bed, an eye mask to shut out what was going on with the other patients on the ward – and also to tell my temporary friends that I was trying to sleep so that they would leave me alone. Writing paper, envelopes and some postage stamps so that I could write a note to those who I did wish to keep in touch with but didn't want to phone. Such a thoughtful idea.

I think back now to a particular friend, who has since passed away, and the effort she made not only to find the hospital but the trouble she had getting there with various obstacles in her way to do with the car, family and a hopeless sense of direction! She brought along some expensive magazines that I would never have bought for myself. She was always available in my times of trouble and we knew that we could call on each other any time of the day or night. I miss her still.

The cards were great to receive, too. Never underestimate what a few written lines of thought can do to help others feel valued. Some of the greetings annoyed me, such as the ones with Christian verses and promises to pray – I was just not in that zone at the time. Yet many people didn't know how I was feeling. From the outside all they knew was that I had cancer and had to undergo some 'terrible' surgery. It was quite possibly more frightening for them to imagine than for me to sleep my way through.

One card arrived and was signed with a single, red heart. My husband's signature emblem. I cried at this one because I was at the stage of thinking that I would just have to get on with life on my own. That's what I wanted to do, but there was a sadness in my musings. No more family Christmases as we had known them and we had shared over thirty together with the children. What if the children got married, had children of their own and when they graduated? How difficult this would all be if I was not with my husband. I needed to give plenty of time to consider all these things.

My sister and her husband wheeled my mother in one day. She was elderly and a little frail, so they asked to borrow a hospital wheelchair and she arrived ceremoniously in said carrier! There was a visitors' room at the end of the ward and I suggested that we all went there. We filled the room as it was rather small but cosy. My mother continued to bemoan as to why two of her daughters had undergone surgery for breast cancer when there was nothing like this in the family that she knew of. Much had changed since she was nursing over half a century ago; life was lived at a much faster pace, there were more chemicals around and also more new, unknown viruses that she had never even heard of. It wasn't until after she passed away that my remaining sister was also diagnosed with breast cancer – three times. Our eldest sister, sadly, died but not until seventeen years after the cancer spread to her liver, and then she battled on for another three years. The determination of the spirit.

As the days passed by and our lymph gland fluid trickled through the tubes into our bags, it was regularly measured. It soon approached the total allotted amount that had to be drained so that we could be discharged. My friend in the bed next to me suggested that we hurried this along a little. I agreed. We moved and we exercised more, as we'd heard that this makes the draining process speed up and we did everything else we could think of to persuade the clear, watery lymph fluid reach that wretched mark on our bags.

Thursday came around and I had been hospitalised for nearly ten days. There was an urgent appointment that I just had to get to the next day. As the measuring nurse approached our beds, my bed neighbour friend and I both made a plea to the staff that we just had to be discharged the next day because of urgent commitments we both had to meet. Fortunately, the line on the bag was reached, our drains were removed and we felt a bit more normal again. We said goodbye to our lovely little bags and I kept it to myself that my urgent appointment was with the hairdresser! People who know me will tell you that I have very thick hair which is quite unmanageable, so I didn't even attempt to wash it while in hospital. Ten days on it wasn't looking its best, even though I tied it up to hide the sad, unruly state it was in.

What a relief when the discharge papers – and more forms – arrived the next day to say that I could go home! Well, at least leave the hospital to move back in with my sister again. Even more relief when she and my brother-in-law came to collect me and drop me immediately at the hairdressers! I apologised to the woman who washed my hair because it was filthy but she was very understanding, thank goodness.

Now I had to get back to as normal as I could and sort out the rest of my life.

chapter four

when it's all over

There is no doubt that, of course, anyone who has had cancer or is living with cancer does change. Their outlook and priorities inevitably change. For me, immediately I left the hospital I wanted to go on a strict diet and examine every ingredient that went into everything I ate. This horrible little 'c' would not be allowed to attack me again. I had too much to do. Too much living, a marriage to sort out, a book to write, two children and a dog to think about. The church would have to wait its turn.

Although I still wanted to be very much left alone, I was beginning to understand that actually we do all need people, each other – my family and friends were more important than I had given them credit for and now it was time to put that right.

Having lived with my sister and brother-in-law for three months it was time to move on. They had been good to me. Not passing any judgement, just being there for me. Not forcing me to go to their church or to engage in any other activity they knew I didn't want to – like praying with them or on my own for that matter. Simple things, like going to the cinema, attending a talk or just going for a walk remained outside the bubble I had built around myself.

A good friend had asked me before Christmas if I'd bought the expensive wool I had my eye on to knit myself a jacket. Of course not, I told her, I won't be able to afford that sort of thing anymore.

Christmas passed through and I saw both my children. It was strange. We went through the motions at my sister's house: dinner, presents, games. They then went home. Back to their father, my husband, my home. Only not with me. Part of me didn't like that. I thought of them altogether, with my dog, and without me. One quite large Christmas bag the children brought with them contained the most beautiful present. The exact knitting yarn I needed to knit the jacket. It cost a lot, I knew that. It was from my husband – just a tag with a red heart confirmed it was from him.

oOoOoOo

Slowly, and I think this is the key to a good recovery, slowly, slowly I managed to find the confidence to move on and move out of my sister's house. I was sleeping so much that most of my time was in or on my bed, but the rest of the time I lived there we all got on well, there was no need to rush my next move. However, I set myself a target of finding my own flat by the end of the year.

It was New Year's Eve when I moved into a small, two bedroom flat close to town. I will never forget that first night when I slept in my own bed in my own home. Although it was on the third floor, I could still hear the parties and the fireworks and the general laughter of people singing in the New Year on the streets outside. I stayed awake in bed until three minutes past twelve. Happy New Year. I felt alone. But wasn't this just what I wanted? Eventually, in the early hours when the noise had died down, I decided to stay in bed and contemplate.

A mattress had been delivered and I had bought some cheap bed linen, so at least I had something to sleep on, but little other furniture. Although I had a small amount of savings, I found that I had to be extremely careful with money and I hadn't had to do that for a long time. I had been fortunate when I was with my husband. Somehow we had always found the money we needed between us. But now it was just me. My sick pay would come to an end in three months' time, so that was the motivation towards my next goal. Get back to work by the end of March. At the beginning of this journey I had told my boss that I would go into hospital, have the op and be back at work before Christmas, totally underestimating how much recovery time I would need. Once anyone starts out on something like this, it's often difficult to accurately estimate just how you're going to feel and exactly how long it's going to take until you feel anything vaguely resembling your 'normal' self – whatever that is.

Older people have told me that everything takes them longer to do and this is exactly how I felt. Shortly after the operation, just having a shower was a lengthy and difficult procedure because the dressing was not to get wet. Lifting my right arm was painful, even though I was keeping up the exercise regime.

I couldn't use the kitchen sink because the plumber was coming on Tuesday to plumb in the washing machine. I didn't have a sofa as the only one I liked the look of was on a four to six week waiting list. I waited. The best place to be was in bed!

Some people find it hard to talk about cancer. My daughter asked me once during a phone call which side 'it' was on, to which I replied, 'the right, thank goodness!' She was puzzled and I explained that if it was on the left it would be nearer my heart, making the operation more dangerous. We discussed if this was the case and she said that she thought our hearts were in the middle of our body. I really don't know if it makes any difference which side the cancer is on and I am sure that the surgeons are really experienced and careful with all the procedures they perform. It was just more of my odd thinking at the time.

A few years later, another close friend had the same diagnosis and she sent me a panic text saying that after her operation she couldn't feel the top of her arm. It was numb. I was not going to lie to anyone and so I told her as it is. The top of my arm is still numb (over ten years later) but why do you need to be able to feel it? You can use the rest of your arm and it doesn't restrict you in any way – as long as you keep doing the exercises so that the muscles in your arm work as best they can.

Another friend had told me that his mother couldn't reach the top shelf in the kitchen after her operation. But then, apparently, she was someone who engaged in self-pity and disabled herself by refusing to get on with life as best she could. Attitude. A lot of what you can get on and do post-op is down to attitude. If you want to be weak and feeble and have people run round after you this may be your prerogative, but if you want to get on, put it behind you and continue living – you can do it!

So here I was, the beginning of a New Year, on my own with everything under my control. It actually felt good for a while. I was on extended sick leave so I concentrated on looking after myself and 'feathering my nest'. The sick leave was probably not at all extended as far as everyone else was concerned, it was just me thinking that I could make a rapid recovery. As I look back on that time now I can't decide if it was just plain selfish or something I needed to do at the time. To be alone, to have no one else to bother about. To suit myself on all fronts. But that was then, what's done is done and I can only reflect on it now and check that over the years I have made peace with those people I offended.

chapter five

looking after yourself

When you live on your own it offers the opportunity to eat what you want, listen to the music you choose, come and go when it suits you and stay in or go out. I made a decision not to have a television in my flat, realising that in the past I had allowed it to waste so much of my time and I didn't want this intrusion any more. This proffered the opportunity for me to read, listen to the radio and best of all – when I was allowed to carry out repetitive movements – knit.

In the UK we are very fortunate to have so many radio stations to listen to and I became friends with several of the people in the serials on offer. Virtual friends, of course. But I came to know them and practised listening to them – after all, they couldn't reply to my comments or answer back! I didn't have much contact with real people; I just needed time to find out who I was, where I was going and to straighten things out in my mind. From the people I have spoken to over the years, it seems that women find it difficult to give themselves permission to look after themselves. Generally they do find it hard to put themselves before others. Joy. That resonated with me at this particular time in my life.

A world of music unlocked itself to me and I began to appreciate the classical melodies that before I wouldn't even bother with. It was nice. Lovely, fine, good, pleasant – all those adjectives sat comfortably with me during the days and evenings on my own. Mozart's operas, concertos and symphonies played their way through my life, as did Schubert's works, together with Bach, Haydn, Chopin and Tchaikovsky. I would definitely recommend all of these and many other classical composers to those recovering from operations and needing rest. To be given the time, the quiet and the uninterrupted peace to just lie on the bed or sit in a comfortable chair to listen and drift along with the rhythm is fantastic. Try it even when it's the last thing you feel like doing. Sit or lie down, close your eyes and just listen to the music, nothing else.

Feeling like a little old lady who revelled in the Classics, I bought myself a small shopping trolley on wheels to complete the appearance. It was a necessity, however, because once a week there was a fresh fruit and vegetable market about fifteen minutes' walk away from my flat. I was determined to eat a healthy, sometimes raw, diet that was rich in the vitamins and minerals my body needed to build up strength, stamina and radiant health. It became a ritual every week. I can't remember which day it was now, but I would take my trolley and buy fruit and veg for the week from the market. It was fairly cheap too. Much less expensive than buying ready-made meals and you know what's gone into it if you make a meal yourself. It took a while for me to get the quantities right and several other people have said this to me, ruing the waste of food when they had bought and cooked too much. Other single friends said that they got used to eating the same meal two, or sometimes three, days in a row. Or you freeze it – this I was not so good at and again had the time to research what could be frozen and how to defrost before it was safe to eat.

I bought a simple, basic food blender from one of the other market stalls – which was indispensable for making smoothies and soups in order to use up the week's fresh food before it went off. No waste meant that I squeezed every last drop of vitamin out of the fruits and composted the skins in a communal bin downstairs.

Because the only time I went out was to the market (and a short walk once a day for fresh air) I wasn't spending much money, which was just as well because my savings were rapidly diminishing and when I returned to work my salary would only just cover rent and bills.

As I've said before, none of us is an island and friends started to ask to meet up with me, take me for lunch or whatever I felt like doing. I put them off as much as I could until I reached a time when it was futile. My excuses ran out and I knew that if I kept repeating the same ones, I would never have any friends left at all. Is that what I really wanted in the end?

A decision to examine my spiritual life found me attending a Sunday sermon at the local church where everyone was very kind and welcoming. Somehow I explained away why I was on my own and that I'd been in hospital. They probably thought I'd had a breakdown or was a substance abuser, but that was ok with me, they could think what they liked; I probably wouldn't see them again. The pastor told anecdotes of times when he had been low, down and out – even in prison, I think I remember – but that God had helped him up and out of the mire. None of us are perfect. After the sermon finished, I drank my Fairtrade coffee, accepted a chocolate biscuit and left with a promise I knew I would break that I would see them next week.

I missed my old church. My ex church? I hadn't been excommunicated yet and I hadn't resigned, so maybe I could still call it 'my church'. But how could I ever go back, especially if my husband was going to be sitting in the next row? It was 'row' because we had got rid of the hard, uncomfortable pews some years previously and replaced them with individual, comfortable chairs which interlocked at the base of their legs. Much better, although there are some who said that we shouldn't be comfortable in church! Anyway, I felt like I'd burnt my bridges there; I couldn't go back as a person who had left their husband and children. I couldn't face them. I knew deep down that what I had done was wrong. Very wrong and unfair. They would be sympathetic, I knew that, but I didn't want sympathy. I don't know what tales they were told, but some of the letters and cards indicated that they were led to believe I had had a breakdown after my operation and was away recuperating. Well, whatever.

My financial situation was worsening so I made a list of all the things I could do to earn some extra money. It was agreed that I could return to work on reduced hours, but that meant reduced pay and I couldn't manage on any less than my full remuneration. What could I manage to do that would bring in a bit more income? Babysitting, knitting, dog walking, cold calling for sales, upmarket escorting... I seriously considered the latter, as long as there was no sex involved. I could accompany people to dinners (I can small talk), on voyages (I love travel) or even to important meetings (I can talk the talk). I once read a book about a woman who did something similar, only her work did involve sex, and she made a good living from this way of life. Her husband never realised what she was doing. I never understood that – how can you live with someone and not know that they drink, gamble, have affairs or whatever and not know? However, a good close friend told me that under no circumstances was I to do that. Somehow she convinced me and I knew, deep down, that really she was right.

Babysitting it was then. I signed up with an agency run by a mother and daughter and I was kept quite busy, especially as I could do Friday and Saturday evenings because I had no social life of my own. I met several lovely families. Most of the children were good. However, this situation broke my heart. What were *my* children doing? Why wasn't I with them? I didn't phone them much because I only had a mobile and it was expensive. We met when we could, but they were both beginning to forge their own lives and, although it was a shock when they found out about my diagnosis, I couldn't see that it affected either of them much. Neither of them wanted me to die and that was about it, but they didn't know how to contribute to keeping me alive. They had their own friends and the rest of the family, some of whom looked out for them, I know.

Chemotherapy was offered, as was radiotherapy and a host of other nicer things that are presented, such as free make-up, exercise classes, endless coffee and cake to help you stay as long as you like to talk. I accepted most of these things – but not the chemo. The medical man – he was a doctor or a surgeon or some kind of specialist, I can't remember exactly now – but he spoke as if he was on commission to get me to agree to the chemotherapy. Blinded with lots of statistics and very few answers to my questions regarding why would anyone want to kill perfectly healthy cells when the nasty 'c' ones had been excavated along with a good margin around the area, I was unsatisfied and unconvinced. When I said that I'd take the radiotherapy but not the chemotherapy, thank you, he still said that he'd give me a couple of weeks to think about it. Frankly, I didn't need a couple of seconds, my mind would not change.

Only a year previously our eldest sister had died after a massive battle against cancer. She had breast cancer seventeen years before and gallantly fought her way back to health. The chemo was so awful for her. It was dreadful for us to watch her going through it, too. The hair loss, the leg ulcers and all the other horrid side effects took a part of her away from us. Her hair grew back and she was so pleased that it was reappearing black and curly, like mine, she would say. But then the nasty little 'c' attacked her liver. She was given eighteen months to live. How can anyone definitively say that? No one knows for sure, no one can predict exactly how long anyone has to live. Three years later she died. I so miss her, even now, my big sister. I told the doc a week later that I definitely refused to have chemo and he *still* asked me if I was sure. Yes. I am sure! My decision. Final answer!

When I eventually got there, the radiotherapy, on the other hand, was quite delightful because I made it into a sort of ritual. I often met another woman at the hospital who was on the same ward as me, with her husband, and we'd have a chat. But I talked as though I was still living with my husband, it felt more respectable and she was an older woman and wouldn't think much of me if I said that I'd left him. Need to be liked. Can't handle criticism at the moment, just need to fit in. Where, I wasn't sure.

So here's the ritual: start with what my mother would call a 'good breakfast'. Healthy fruit smoothie, porridge or cereal, toast or crisp bread, shower and spray with something that smells lovely, dress in pretty underwear and smart clothes – including heels. Make-up and hair done, leave the flat ready to take on the world. At the hospital, speak to and smile at everyone in the waiting room, they may need a bit of encouragement. Undress in a too small cubicle and put on a gown that (thank goodness) opens at the front in a modest cross-over fashion. When name is called, enter room and lie on cold trolley bed and stay really, really still. There was always some soothing music playing through the speakers at just the right volume, too. Everyone else leaves the room and it's just me and the most beautiful, emerald green laser beam that appears to hover above me on the ceiling. Two minutes later everyone bustles in and someone says, "That's it for today, then. See you tomorrow."

I reverse the preparation processes mentioned above and take myself off to a lovely tea room for an exotic coffee and cake. There I read a magazine or paper that's in the rack and then have a wander round a few shops. Depending on how tired I was feeling, I would either go home and have a rest on the bed or stay out a bit longer. Occasionally I would meet a friend to share the coffee/cake part, but I usually preferred to go it alone. And that was my routine every day for five days until it finished five weeks later. The hospital staff didn't work weekends so we got Saturdays and Sundays off too. I had my last radiotherapy session, gave the staff a tin of biscuits and hoped it had all been worth it. It was the end of February; I needed to get back to work.

My time of living in a recuperation bubble was coming to an end and I felt scared of what was going to happen next. I accepted an invitation from my husband to go somewhere for a drink with him and we talked about what had happened and what the future held in store for both of us. Together or not. We exchanged pleasantries and talked about the children and the dog and a lot of other things we used to share together.

Looking back, I suppose I was depressed and in a state where I couldn't work out what I wanted, but I knew that whatever it was, it would have to be forever. I couldn't go through another relationship break-up, so it was 'until death us do part' or divorce and no going back. The finality of the decision to be made was overwhelming.

I found a therapist, negotiated a fee I could afford and attended weekly sessions. How was I feeling? How *was* I feeling? How was *I* feeling? How was I *feeling*? Whatever way it was asked, I just didn't know but was forced to say something. So we looked at the pros and cons of marriage reconciliation and generally how to find out what I wanted in life. My therapist would then 'give me the tools to go out and get it'. She helped me to build back up my self-confidence and I saw more opportunities. Possibilities that perhaps had always been there but not so obvious before.

The days were filled with more activity as I prepared to return to the workforce. I walked a couple of dogs for their owner who had sprained her ankle, I babysat and got paid for it, I looked after another dog while the owner worked a long day and did various other bits and pieces to help me feel slightly more useful.

Energy levels rose as I exercised, ate properly, started to interact more with other people and regularly took multivitamins and a tonic. Our mother spent her ninety first birthday in hospital recovering from a stroke. My sister and I found a suitable care home and moved her in when she was strong enough. Two years later she died in her sleep and the loss was deeply saddening, reviving all the other memories of loss – including my lump, strangely enough – my sister, father (who passed away when I was twelve) and my marriage. But had I actually lost the latter or was it just in hibernation?

Despite the fact that I thought I was living a healthy life, my stomach didn't agree. I felt like buying shares in Imodium. The GP sent me to the hospital for an endoscopy, not pleasant but after what I had been through it was bearable. They found an ulcer. There's a surprise. Life throws things at you, and always will, but there is only so much you can take – however positive a personality you may be blessed with, stress and strain will reveal itself somewhere, somehow in your body. But it is our response to life traumas that help us to be strong and get through them. The ulcer medication was fantastic. It mended or covered or did whatever it was meant to do and I could once again eat fairly normally. More importantly, I found that I was able to go out and not worry about where the nearest WC was located. Marvellous.

The medics also decided that my blood pressure was too high. It's always been high. So I was fitted with a twenty-four hour monitor involving small pads, wires and a box. Every so often (I think it must have been about once an hour) the box part would inflate slightly and click, sending a reading back to base. This wasn't too inconvenient apart from a meeting I had to attend with staff and students at the college where I worked. In case the machine went off during a pregnant pause in the meeting, I thought it prudent to say at the beginning what may happen should the contraption inflate. Most people didn't notice but the two students did and sniggered to themselves. In a nice way, they just thought the whole thing was very amusing. I returned their looks with a smile and continued with the meeting.

chapter six

time to come home...

The days and weeks meandered through my life as I kept pace with my spending, sleeping and eating to make sure everything was in order and nothing was out of place, so that I could look back on this time and know that I had done the right thing. It probably wasn't and isn't the right thing to do, but it was done now and I had to think about what may happen next.

Among the pleasant, but I felt unnecessary, cards and letters I received during my recuperation were two quite horrid letters. Both from relatives. I think that they were just expressing their hurt at our marriage break-up but they kept coming to mind as I tried to forget the accusing words. One was quite directive, ordering me to go back to my husband and children. Another was very accusing in telling me that I didn't realise how lucky I was with a husband like mine and that she could only imagine what it must be like to have someone who loved her so much. She was in an unhappy, almost abusive relationship and I presume couldn't bring herself to accept that I had something better than that and I was choosing to leave it.

I heard through my mother-in-law that my husband had taken the children to a Greek island. We used to holiday somewhere in the Mediterranean every summer with the children. The pang of regret and sadness hit me hard in the middle of my heart. I had to go out there, I had to find my family and tell them all that it had all been a terrible mistake; I was ill and didn't know what I was doing. Then my husband would take me back and we could all resume a 'normal' life.

Mother-in-law was at my (ex?) home, so I phoned and said that I had to come over and see her. Being a very reasonable person, she agreed to meet me. It was awkward when I first arrived in the house that I had left over six months previously, but for the first time I was able to put into words how I was really feeling and what I wanted to happen in the not too distant future. I begged her to tell me where they were staying and said that I would take the next flight out to meet with them. As I said, she was a very reasonable person and made no verbal judgement about what I intended to do. She wanted to see us back together, so maybe she thought that it would have to happen whichever way it would.

Without giving much thought to the implications, I booked the flight and hoped that I could sleep on the floor of the apartment where my family were staying. If not, then I would check into another hotel along the road. Once I had the tickets, I thought that I'd better phone my husband to let him know I was coming out.

It was a strange and strained telephone conversation, which went along the lines of me saying that I was coming to see him, him replying that he wasn't even in the UK, me responding that I knew and I had my plane tickets and him finishing the conversation by asking what time my flight landed and that they would pick me up from the airport in a jeep they'd hired. I'm not sure that he was surprised, actually.

At the very beginning of our relationship, over forty years ago, he asked me if I wanted to go away for the weekend along the coast with him, Although I agreed, he said something – I truly forget what it was now – that made me so enraged, I refused to go at the last minute. He went alone. A couple of days later, I changed my mind and took a train to the place he was staying. I would turn up, knock on the door and ask his forgiveness that I had been so horrid, but that it was called for under the circumstances. He would understand and take me into his arms and eventually his bed. So I thought...

On that occasion, I had to phone him because when I arrived at the location I found that it was fairly remote and there were no taxis. Can you believe it – no taxis?! There was no option but for me to phone and ask if he could pick me up. That phone conversation was similar to the one I have just described when he was in Crete. He asked me how I was, I replied fine, he then asked me where I was, to which my reply of *actually just five miles away from him* caught him by surprise. He did drive out to collect me and the rest is history, as they say.

So, back on the Greek island, they arrived at the airport in an old, battered jeep which apparently had just taken them on a tour of the island. We went back to the apartment and my husband promptly ignored me. It was getting late and as dark as it does out there, so I thought that I'd better broach the subject of where I could sleep. *Not in my bed* was his reply, so I gathered together some blankets and a spare pillow to make up a bed on the balcony and slept under the stars. Neither of the children offered to give up their bed for me, so I guess they were as mad at me as he was.

It was a bit hard sleeping on the ground, but I felt that I deserved it and the starlit night was something so wonderful that I'm glad I managed the entire night out in the open. The temperature wasn't that cold either, so I was fine.

In the morning, my husband got up and ignored everyone else. I tried to talk to my daughter and my son separately. They seemed more understanding of what I had done than I expected. I attempted a conversation with my husband as he lay on the sunbed. This was more difficult than I had anticipated and I decided to give up. I went into the apartment, lay on his bed and wept. My daughter was very sweet and tried to comfort me, but she was young and had experienced little of life and love and boyfriends. However, I think that she wanted her mum and dad to reconcile, so we talked about what could happen.

If my husband wouldn't even talk to me, I didn't know what I could do towards any attempt at reconciliation. I was only going to be there for three days, so there was little time to lose. I had a three-day return ticket and so there had to be a lot of fast discussion about our future.

Eventually, on his terms and in his time, he agreed that we should take a walk without the children. In the holiday surroundings and sunshine beating down on the olive groves, I think that we actually fell in love again. As soppy as it sounds, I believe this is what happened. Not without hurtful exchanges, though. To exchange some home truths is not an easy process, but if this marriage was to stand any chance of survival, some things had to be said.

I'd read before – and we had been told on a marriage course we went through together several years earlier – that it was better to talk and find a solution, rather than bury hurts. I hadn't done this before. I was like my father; when he was alive my mother could get away with anything. He never complained or picked a fight, he always felt that life was too short for wars so he went along with anything for a quiet life. I was twelve when he died and all these years later I miss him and wonder what he would have thought of not only what I had done, but how he would have got on with his grandchildren. These days he would have had a great granddaughter. It would have been so interesting to observe their interactions. But he's gone and we can't bring him back, only the memories that are held close to the heart.

In order to not 'let the sun go down on an argument' my husband and I thrashed out a few things that we had never talked about before. I cried, he held me and we all went for dinner as a family that night. It was good.

The following day went by far too quickly, it was just too short. The familiarity of each other and everyone together as a proper family felt right and I knew that I would have to make a momentous decision. Then I would have to encourage my husband to agree!

When they all came with me to the airport I felt that it was to say goodbye for the very last time. Never again would I have to go through this separation. Nor would they.

Leaving the warm, sunny climate and returning to a wet, damp UK on my own wasn't easy. I entered my empty, cold flat and tried to warm up by putting the heating on full blast, making a hot chocolate and wrapping myself in the duvet. It was a bit of a Bridget Jones moment, but I knew that once the rest of my family were back in the UK things would change for the better. I counted the days and hours until they returned and we could have another conversation about getting back together again.

Sometimes life doesn't pan out as we expect it to and this can be for an unknown reason. I think that we can all learn from mistakes, events and things that don't seem to go quite right – or as we sometimes tell ourselves how it should be. It doesn't always go according to our time scale, either. Patience. A great gift.

Once my husband and family were back in the UK I had hoped that we would meet up again soon. I had hoped that I would be able to move back to the family home soon. But it didn't work like that.

We sometimes play games with each other, knowingly or unknowingly. I knew that my husband had been hurt really badly and I needed to make it up to him. But he also wanted to be in control of our future, I could see that. I had no option but to wait.

I phoned a lifelong friend who lived miles away in the north of the country and asked her what I should do. *He'll come round* she told me. But when he didn't *come round* in my time scale, I began to feel sad, afraid and a little bit of giving up crept into my thinking.

It's a good job my friend and I both had free minutes on our mobiles because we spent a long time each evening talking about possible scenarios and how I could approach my husband. He was still my husband, after all. She eventually made contact with him and he thought I was with someone else. How could that be? I'd just flown over fifteen hundred miles to be with him for three days, wearing my heart on my sleeve. Didn't that count for anything?

I made several abortive attempts at writing a letter to him. We used to write cards and notes to each other when we were together before, but this one had to be word perfect. Finally, I settled on an effort that I thought explained how I felt and would reach out to him and maybe even pull at his heart strings. I posted it on Thursday.

By the following Wednesday I was speaking on the phone again with my girlfriend who assured me that he was not going to be rushed into taking me back. She had spoken with him on the phone to try and gain an understanding of what was going on in his mind. This was a useful tactic as he asked her how I was doing and she was able to tell him how much I missed him and my home. I'd said this to him in my letter, but she confirmed it to him verbally.

A few more weeks passed by and I heard nothing from my husband. The problem is, and we probably all know this, men and women think very differently over certain (and maybe many) subjects. Furthermore, when we try to guess what each other is thinking it often compounds the issue and results in drastic miscommunication. I was beginning to think that the plans for reconciliation as I understood them were thwarted and it was never going to happen. As a result, I started to get on with my life. I continued to eat healthily, exercise and knit. My sleeping pattern settled into a routine that meant I felt better and more alive during the day. I made contact with some old friends and went to the cinema, theatre, exhibitions – anything that offered a free or reduced entrance fee, as I still had to watch the money. People came to supper or lunch, which was good, but I appreciated my solitude once they had gone. Perhaps we weren't meant to get back together at all. Maybe this is how it would be for the rest of my life. Maybe.

Plunging into work life, I often worked late and sometimes took work home but I was very aware that I couldn't return to the negative work/life balance I had before my diagnosis. Whether this was a contributory factor or not, I will never know, but my suspicion was that it could well have been. I saw my children and dog now and again, but they were more and more building their own lives.

Although my husband told me that I was not to go to the house, he didn't realise that I still had a back door key. In those days no one locked the back gate. I really wanted to stand in the house to see how I felt. One day I did just that. Knowing he was out at a meeting I entered through the back gate and back door and was greeted by the dog. What a lovely moment, but his water bowl was empty and he hadn't been brushed for a long time, his coat was matted and he generally didn't look very good. I filled his water bowl and he drank thirstily for quite a while. I brushed his coat and cleaned his face and eyes. We sat together on the floor until I had to leave. I didn't want to be accused of breaking into my own house. It was clear that no one was coping; the pile of ironing and washing up, empty boxes and rubbish bin that was full to overflowing. I just knew that my place was there and I had to try harder to convince my husband that I needed to get back home. To him, to the family, to the dog and to our family home.

I cried all the way back to my flat, about eight miles away, and as I put the key in the communal door and then into my own front door, I realised that this wasn't my home. I shouldn't be here on my own.

I phoned him that night and asked if we could meet, but his response was *why?* I said that we needed to sort things out, to which he replied that there was nothing to sort out and that I needn't think that I was going to go straight back home as if nothing had happened. I would have to wait.

So wait, I did. My patience was tested.

A week later I received a text saying that he was ready to meet me.

It was a lovely, crisp, autumnal day as we walked alongside a small stream under the arched trees. As it was a Saturday, there were several families out together and this saddened me to see them getting on with their lives and us wasting ours. We talked. That was good because I managed to say once again how I saw things – which were not always the same as he saw them, but on most issues we found common ground. He told me that if I ever, ever left him again it would definitely be the last time and he would no way even think about having me back. I said that I wouldn't put us both through this again.

After that afternoon, another week went by with no communication.

Then I received the most beautiful card through the post containing simple words, 'Time to come home' and signed with the familiar red heart.

Needless to say, I cried again, but this time they were tears of joy. But I was also confused – how, when would I go home? Now, next week, next year? I thought I'd better leave it a couple of days and phoned my girlfriend to see what she thought. Again, looking back, I couldn't seem to make my own decisions. I thought I had become independent and strong, but the big things in life, like repairing a marriage, were difficult to organise.

Somehow we sorted it out between us. I gave notice to my landlord, packed up my things and moved back home. During my 'sabbatical' as we came to refer to it as, I had bought things like a bed, sofa, clothes airer, kettle, crockery and other furniture.

51

Consequently, back home we found ourselves with two of many things! There was a lot of reorganisation of furniture and sending things to the charity shops that went on, but it all settled down after a while.

One of my neighbours asked me straight if I was back for good now. I replied in the affirmative. They had been good to my husband while I was gone and it felt a bit like a reprimand. Deserved, of course.

Sometimes it felt like we were starting all over again, but it wasn't, we'd spent over twenty-five years living together and knew each other's ways, but I suppose we both wanted it to work this time and had to tread carefully until we were once again a fully established couple.

Most people were kind. Some invited us to their house and we tried to act as normally as possible, skirting around the reason I had left, in fact not even mentioning that I'd been away. It was difficult at times because I wanted to talk about museums I'd visited, my trip to the Isle of Wight, exhibitions that I found interesting – but all these things I had done on my own and I didn't want others to think that I'd had a good time. Because a lot of the time I was heartbroken. I had to go into therapy. It wasn't easy, but then I suppose it wasn't easy for him either. I had grown up. Not sure how much, but a change had happened in me and I wanted to keep it that way.

chapter seven

a word on faith

The other aspect of my life that had to be addressed – no, correction, I wanted to address – was that of my spiritual life. I had turned my back on everything when I left home, including my church and God.

I had belonged to our church since the children were small. It was local, the women were nice and friendly and I thought it would be good for the children to make new friends and learn a solid base on which to build their lives. Back then, they also offered a 'Shoppers' Crèche' once a week, which offered me an invaluable hour and a half to be child free. At this time, our daughter had started her first school and our son was just a baby, so he benefitted in the Shoppers' Crèche from the interaction with other babies. The women were not only kind, but they were gentle too and this gave me confidence that our son would be well looked after. Eventually, I got it down to a fine art – drop him off at the crèche, dash round the supermarket, back home, put the kettle on while I emptied the bags and filled the cupboards with food shopping and then got on with the Open University degree course I had embarked on and finally back to pick him up before they finished. You don't get much free time when you are a mother with young children.

One thing, among many, my husband is actually good at, is encouraging me to do what I really wanted. Because of that I felt that I couldn't fail. So when I said that I was nowhere bright enough to do a *degree* course and he said *of course you are* it made me think that perhaps I could be. This happened over thirty-five years ago but I clearly remember the day after giving birth to our daughter, sitting up in my hospital bed trying to finish off an OU assignment. My graduation was a lovely day with both my sisters and mother attending; now I look back at that photograph of the four of us and sadly miss two influential women in my life. My eldest sister died first and then a few years later, Mother.

It was time now to make an appointment to visit our pastor,

say I was sorry and ask if I could come back into the fold. He didn't give me a particularly easy time, either, but it taught me the gravity of the action I had taken. Loving, kindness and forgiveness were all there, but I felt like I had to earn it. Maybe that's right, too. But you never have to earn God's love, forgiveness and affection, it's always there but we have to recognise it.

For me, it was present in the friend I made at the hospital, the nurses, every one of the cards and letters I received, the pastor at the church I visited and everywhere around – if only I'd looked and seen. But I was too wrapped up in my own determination to forge a life for myself on my own.

To believe in God is an ongoing process and a two-way one. He will speak to you, but you have to listen. He will provide the way for you, but you have to want to open the door, and most of all He will never give you a burden that is too much to bear. He teaches us through life experiences and He guides us through His word, the Bible. But I had to do my part and I realised that I had gone AWOL – in other words, absent without official leave.

The cards I received from other Christians contained verses of scripture, but the way I was feeling at the time meant that they fell on deaf ears. I didn't believe they were true anymore. Now I see things very differently.

When people have an accident or are absent from church for a while with a disease or some other life trauma, the response of the congregation varies. The response of the individual varies, too. I know of another person who 'fell away' and on her return, she wanted balloons, banners and trumpets to sound out her return. I didn't. I wanted to quietly slip into the pew and not be noticed. However, when something major like a separation happens, one's absence does get noticed. My husband had kept the faith while I was gone and had attended church on his own. People notice when suddenly you appear without your spouse. Of course they do. People want to help. They want to make it better. It's a natural, human response.

The first time I re-entered the church doors after my absence, clutching my husband's arm, I felt exposed, frightened and worried about what people would think of me. I didn't need to worry. Most people were welcoming and acted as if I'd never left. Those who didn't know what to say just kept their distance. Forgiveness. It needs practice. God forgives our sins over and over again, but people still need to be reminded of His grace that we can all have, it just needs digging up sometimes for certain situations. Every word of that first sermon was directed at me. It was! It was one of those times when I felt that I was wretched, but also loved and cared for by people, by God and by His angels that he sends in human form.

I had fallen away and followed my own, selfish ideas of how I wanted my life to be, but then I came to a realisation that it wasn't what I wanted at all. Non-believers have suggested to me that we can all do what we like, say we're sorry to God and carry on regardless if He is a forgiving God. It doesn't really work like that. The Christian faith has to be worked at and the Bible tells us how to do this, as well as giving us guidelines for a purposeful and fruitful life.

'... For I know the plans I have for you,' declares the Lord, 'plans to prosper you and not to harm you, plans to give you hope and a future...' This verse can be found in Jeremiah 29 verse 11. This was written for everyone.

However, He also gave each one of us free will and this can be exercised in whatever way we like, if we want to. For those who follow God and do not swerve from the narrow path, I take my hat off because it is a really difficult thing to do. Every single day we are faced with temptations and decisions. Some are obviously right and others are obviously wrong; for others we have to seek guidance. I used to have trouble with discipline, being told what to do and how to do it.

These days I have come to realise that actually the Ten Commandments form the baseline of how we are to live our lives to keep us safe and prosper. I think that I always knew that deep down inside, when I came out of my 'sabbatical', I had to revisit these guidelines for living properly:

1   Put God first (thou shalt have no other gods before me).
2   Don't worship idols (thou shalt not make any graven image

and worship it).

3   Use God's name with respect (do not take the name of the Lord your God in vain).
4   Don't work on a Sunday unless you really have to (remember the Sabbath Day and keep it holy).
5   Respect your parents (honour your Father and your Mother).
6   Don't kill anyone (thou shalt not kill).
7   Be faithful in marriage (thou shalt not commit adultery).
8   Don't take anything that's not yours unless you have permission to do so (you shall not steal).
9   Don't lie (you shall not bear false witness against your neighbour).
10   Don't be envious of others (you shall not covet your neighbour's house, wife or anything that is your neighbour's).

These are worth dwelling on. They appear in Exodus chapter 20, but also if you search the Internet you will find variations. Some more modern than others. However, if this is all too much to follow, they have been condensed into two main rules which say something along the lines of *Love God with all your heart and love others as much as you love yourself*.

Imagine if everyone loved one another, then there wouldn't be any killing, disrespect, stealing, lying or envy. We'd all get along together and help each other. Isn't that how we would all love to live? Less strains and stresses for the individual and a lot less wars.

There's a certain feeling when you drop a piece of cutlery in a restaurant, answer a quiz question wrongly, shout out at someone you misidentify – a feeling of being the centre of attention. All eyes on you. Blood rushing to the head and especially the cheeks, going red. Well, this was how I felt that first time I returned to church. It was probably the embarrassment of my sins, but God and true Christians don't judge, don't condemn but simply loved me back into the church family.

It took a few weeks for me to feel comfortable again and many questions of how I was feeling now. Was I supposed to say that I was better? Everything's alright now? Thanks, but I'm fine? I said exactly what I felt and those who wanted to take me aside to either find out more, give me a telling off or attempt to help me feel more at ease, were all treated the same as far as I was concerned. Some of us are more curious than others. Some were able to just leave the details alone and continue from where we left off.

On reflection, it was the little things that I was scared about – did I look ok? How much should I put in the offering? Shall I make notes? Are my heels too high? In the end we have to reach the point where we're comfortable in our own skin and I wonder if that only comes with maturity. Age. It can also arrive when you truly know God, our Lord and Saviour, because to Him you look great all the time. He made each one of us, whether you believe it or not, He did.

One evening a bit later on, I decided to go to the evening service at our church. My husband never went to that one, he still doesn't, but I wanted to sit in a contemplative space. However, when I arrived, I just didn't know where to sit. If I sat on my own, people would wonder if I was really back for good. They may also be pointing the finger and think that I had no friends to come back to (my irrational thoughts). But what if I sat next to someone who would prefer I didn't sit next to them? What is the worst that could happen? Actually no one snubs you or is horrible to you in church, generally, that is. All of these potential scenarios I was getting all worked up about were in my mind. Would I do that to someone? Would I play my part in forgiving others' sins? Now, I hope I would and I certainly would welcome people back into the church with open arms. That's exactly what happened to me and it is a good model that I now follow.

So I sat on my own a few seats in from the edge, and as other people turned up, some sat next to me on my right and some to my left. In fact, I was flanked by two of the most honest, upright and loving women I know – and I felt comfortable. Reassured. Loved.

Of course, the sermon was directed at only me! The words of the preacher hit home and I felt a little uneasy, but God (through the speaker) disciplines those He loves and I sat there that evening and took my discipline, as it was precisely what I deserved.

Another thing about God is that not only does He give you what you can manage, if He gives you a situation that you feel you absolutely can't manage, He will give you the courage, help, people, scriptures, time, love or whatever you need to get through. If you believe.

The story of the Prodigal Son comes to mind, especially the part when the father comes running to meet his lost son. Never mind the ring on his finger and the finest robes and the feast, but just the fact that he moved towards his son, and quickly at that, to show how happy he was to have him back in the family.

I was fortunate. My husband, my family, my church and God all welcomed me back and I never want to go away again. The Christian life isn't always easy, no one ever promises that, but if you are faithfully seeking the right way to live, it's all written down in the Bible. Put others first, love your enemy – if everyone did that in the world it would see an end to all wars. And be true to yourself. You know if you've done something wrong, said a hateful word, refused to forgive someone. It keeps you awake at night, it lays in your thinking throughout the day and it will be in your memory until you do something about it. There were several people I needed (wanted) to see to ask their forgiveness. It wasn't easy. Some made light of it and others put it down to me not being well. I wasn't well, I'd had a big operation, but that was no excuse to hurt people the way I did.

One woman took me to a lovely tea room on a bright sunny day and told me that she didn't want details but she just wanted to know how to pray for me. That meant a lot. When people pray for you it has the most amazing effect. There's one song we sing in church that says Our Saviour (God) can move the mountains. I felt like I had a lot of mountains to move to reach those I wanted to reconcile my friendship with. God made this happen in the most amazing ways. Slowly, I was approached to see if I would go on various different rotas. That helped me to fit in and feel more like one of the church family once again. People were very kind. We were invited to dinner, teas and other events as a couple once again.

Now, ten years on, I still worship at the same church. A

different pastor had now taken over from the previous one who retired. He wouldn't have seen or maybe not even heard all this that had been going on with me and my husband. Maybe he does know, maybe he doesn't. Either way, it has no bearing on how I am now. I worship, serve and hopefully am of some help to other people. Especially those who have had a diagnosis of breast cancer, and in every congregation there will be a few. More if it's a large church.

To the Christians I say, *hold on to your faith*, to the unbelieving searcher I say, *cast your worries and your cares on Christ – He will not let you down*. A friend once said to me, "Well He hasn't let us down so far!" And He never will.

Many of us will know or at least have heard what is termed *The Lord's Prayer*. Here's my interpretation. Again, depending on where you stand at this point in time, you may concur with some of what I'm saying or you may dismiss it. We all have free will and options to our own and others' opinions about everything.

Our Father who art in Heaven

I believe that we all have a Spiritual Father who lives in Heaven and I therefore believe that there is such a place as 'Heaven'. My Spiritual Father lives in Heaven, but also in me by means of the Holy Spirit and is therefore my protector in times of trouble.

Hallowed be thy Name

I've always thought of 'hallowed' as meaning the same as sacred. The God I believe in is a sacred being and therefore His name is hallowed.

Thy Kingdom Come

I know it's an old-fashioned term, but 'thy' simply means 'your' and if this is the way it was originally written then don't get wound up about it. Your Kingdom Come – I would love the Lord's Kingdom to reign on Earth while I was still alive, and this may happen, but by expressing this in a prayer it just makes it a bit more real.

Thy Will Be Done on Earth as it is in Heaven

Whatever God's will is, I want it to be done on this Earth. In Heaven, all the Ten Commandments are adhered to (and therefore there is no pain, suffering or war) and we have the capacity to create this peace on Earth. If only more people would believe and follow the Bible's guidelines...

Give us this day our daily bread

Simply put, give us enough to eat on a daily basis. Whatever our daily amount or portion is: enough so that we don't starve but not so much that we become gluttonous or overweight or wasteful of that which is left over.

Forgive us our trespasses...

Forgive our sins, our wrongdoings. None of us can live a perfect life coming up to the standards that God sets for us. We may try but we cannot do this every minute of our lives. We are human and we make mistakes. Sometimes we reflect on responses we have made and wish we'd said or done something differently. This is being human. Only God is perfect. He will forgive us and so will others, usually, if we ask for their forgiveness.

...as we forgive those who trespass against us

We would do well to cultivate a forgiving attitude towards others from the small things like when someone else takes our parking space to the bigger things, and you can think of your own examples here. When we bear a grudge against someone who has committed an act of depravity against us or our family, it eats away at us. When we forgive that person, we are relieved, as they are, so the relationship is restored. I believe that this is even more important within families as well as within the church family and especially with others outside the church.

Lead us not into temptation but deliver us from evil

This is a big one. How often during the day are we tempted?

More importantly, how often do we recognise temptation and make the right decision to avoid a wrongful act? Very often, I suspect. I know that during my lifetime I have been tempted many times. Before I became a Christian I often gave into things that I fundamentally knew to be wrong, but I ploughed on through anyway. Now there is no excuse. As mentioned before, we have been given the guidelines for living by the Ten Commandments, so when confronted with a temptation and a decision to make, see if the outcome lines up with these. We will be tested in this life but it's our response to the test that will make us the character that we are and if we want to be better then it's up to us to try harder and ask for help. Help comes in so many forms: through people, through reading the Bible, through prayer and through talking to God. I have often prayed, 'Lord, I don't know what to do, please help me.' Some people are given visions, I'm not one of them but I have had dreams that seem to fit with the problem at the time. It's interesting to make a dream journal. I kept one for many years, and looking back it is fascinating to see how a dream has become a reality later on, or has indeed been the guidance I was looking for at the time.

The Bible also tells us that God will not tempt us beyond what we can handle, but this is often interpreted that we can handle all things with God. We will be led into temptation, but we will be given the way through and out of it. So we have to go through certain challenging situations. Sometimes it is to help us understand and to help us grow as a person and as a Christian. When evil is coming at us, we are to depend on God. He will 'deliver' us from evil, but it may not be via the route we expect. Sometimes we have to go down another road to find out a bit more about ourselves, about others, about God.

For Thine is the Kingdom, the Power and the Glory, for ever and ever.

The greatness and the power and the glory belong to God and He has the power over all our kingdoms, although there are those who will not believe that and prefer an alternative faith. The Lord made this world and everything in it, so it belongs to Him and He is entitled to the glory and power over everything.

Amen

Meaning 'so be it', this word indicates the end of a prayer. Everything that has been prayed up until this final word is agreed by those who have prayed or have listened to a prayer and agree with it.

This is such a clever and useful prayer that if you never pray anything else it will cover everything!

At the time of my cancer diagnosis, I called out to God 'Why?' When my sister was diagnosed for the third time with cancer, she struggled to understand His plan. At the time our elder sister was taken from this earth, we wept and asked God 'Why?' To some it may seem a bit of a diversion to say that we don't understand the ways of God and that He has a plan for all our lives, it's just that we can't always see it. We certainly can't see the future like He does. But at the end of the day, and I have often heard my sister say this, we cannot know the plans He has made for our lives, but we have to be content to know that He is in control and will not let us down.

chapter eight

looking to the future

I am not in remission, I don't live with cancer but I will acknowledge that I *had* cancer and I don't have it any more. Yes, it may come back, yes it may spread, but you can't think like that and live your life in a way that is so cautious you don't do any living. That's my take on it all, anyway. Accept each day as it comes. Every morning I wake up and thank God that he has brought me safely through the night and I submit each day to Him. It's amazing what opportunities He will open up for you. If you don't already belong to a church, I would urge you to visit one. Just to see. And be open to what God wants to show you or have you do.

Some people think that Christians live a dull life. This couldn't be further from the truth. The Bible advises and guides, but God also gives us free will. That's often where we go wrong! But He has a huge heart and always the willingness to forgive our mistakes if we are repentant. I have been along some dark roads, not only during the past ten years, but generally during the whole of my life. Some things I have done were not only unforgivable but downright dangerous. I don't dwell on these now; I know I have been forgiven, baptised as an adult and am free from condemnation. So no matter what people may say, as long as I know that I'm right in God's eyes is actually all that matters now. He didn't prevent my cancer because I had lessons to learn while I was going through it and they were all good life lessons.

My husband and I are fully involved with our church. We take our turn on certain rotas, but again we both need to be careful not to take on too much. I've overdone it before and don't intent to return to those circumstances. We're both getting older by the day and that's true of everyone. The only certainty in life is that we are born and we die, so what we do with the time in between is up to us as individuals. No one can *make* you do anything. You always have the last word with your life, with your body, with the drugs you take or refuse to take.

I have recently become interested in Mindfulness and I find that this is helpful in every aspect of life. To take the time literally to smell the coffee is to be recommended. Life has taken on a speed of its own, with new technology and remote controls. We no longer have to be in the same place to make something happen. You can operate your washing machine, house lights and curtains when you are not at home via a remote control, should you so wish. A text message to let someone know you are thinking of them at a difficult time is instant. We no longer have to wait for the post to take one to three days to deliver a handwritten card or letter. Although, in certain circumstances, I still do so out of choice. It is sometimes nice to receive a thoughtful card that is sent to cheer.

The development of technology is to be applauded. It's progress. It's development and we all need to either take part and go along with it or we will be swept along with it. As I'm writing this now, I have a heavy cold and a really bad ear ache. So I looked on the Internet and found out what is wrong – inner ear infection, which will go of its own accord within a week. Usually caused by vestibular neuritis and labyrinthitis, apparently. I always look at more than one source of medical information, so another site suggested that I rest and remain immobilised, avoiding bright lights. And another to put a warm cloth against the ear, and that really, really helped!

However, if I couldn't have looked this up immediately I would have asked my husband to take me to the Accident and Emergency Department of our local hospital, waited there for several hours and be told the same things. So although some of us don't like computers (I only don't when they go wrong and that's often because I've given it the wrong command), if we embrace change, go with it, find out what we need to know so that we can work things out, it could well be to our advantage.

Incidentally, a day later, having followed the instructions from my 'internet doctor' by taking some pain killers and placing a warm cloth on the painful ear, I feel a lot better already. I'm just saying that I think we should question, research and make informed decisions on medical issues.

Please don't misunderstand me. I have the highest regard for doctors, nurses, surgeons, in fact everyone who works in the medical field. Like many other people, I have also given birth to two healthy children, undergone a hysterectomy, tonsillectomy, nose operation (not cosmetic, by the way) and several other minor procedures within the NHS and I have nothing but praise for the way I was treated and the manner in which I recovered. Along with my surviving sister, we have seen our eldest sister, mother, father-in-law, mother-in-law, uncle and several friends pass away from this earth because there was nothing else that could be done for them medically. I have seen life and death. While I'm alive on this earth, I try to motivate and encourage others to live well and show them how to be grateful. The rest is up to the individual.

None of us can know for sure what life holds for us or what is just around the corner. I remember a time many years ago when I had to attend an interview for a job that I had been doing for about a year. There was one post and two of us applying for it. I knew, just knew that I would get it. I was younger, smarter and had more forward-thinking ideas than the other person who was pleasant enough, but a little staid in her ways and close to retirement. She had a very basic idea of how to operate a word processor and I often had to show her how to perform a function with certain keys. They gave the job to her.

It was like a slap in the face, not only was I redundant with a young family that needed my income as well as my husband's, but I was just not prepared for this outcome. However, my situation meant that I had to attend the local Job Centre, stand in line (it was that long ago – not like the current day when everything is done online) and report in regularly until I could find a job. It only took a few weeks, but it showed me how some people's lives are dependent on others to allow them to have some money to buy food. I was also led into a job where I stayed for ten years and had the opportunity to work my way up to a respectable level and salary.

Whatever comes along may knock us back, but it's our determination and doggedness that will get us through. Learn how to pick yourself up, dust yourself off and start all over again as the song goes. Allow yourself the time to cry, mourn and worry – but make it time limited! At some point you have to get on or you will drown in misery, boredom, self-pity, resentment or whatever you feel. At the end of the day, it's up to you. Gather round you people who are positive, whether that's on Facebook or Twitter (yes, even at my age I tweet). Surround yourself with posters, stickers or whatever that carries a motivational sentence, a famous quote or a saying that you find helpful. If you've never found one then carry out a search on the Internet. Don't have a computer? Go to your local library, ask a friend or save up for one. There is always a way through. Break down those barriers and even if you haven't ever tried something before, have a go. Ask yourself what's the worst that could happen? And you'll probably find that it never does, or at least it doesn't happen as badly as you imagined. If you really don't like something you've tried for the first time then don't do it again! You have choice. We all have choice.

When I look to my future, our future, I know full well that it probably won't be as I would ideally like it to be. We're edging towards retirement age but still have debts to pay off and an adult son who lives with us. Fortunately, my husband enjoys his work and refuses to retire. So if you do love your job, no one is going to force you to retire. He asked me what he would do if he did retire, but my list of jobs didn't quite persuade him! I may not become a famous author with all of my books selling at a rate of knots so that we don't have to worry about income, but that thought doesn't stop me writing.

I would encourage you to look at what sort of future you would like. Then look at what you have already and see if it's feasible to fill (or bridge) the gap. Perhaps it isn't. Are you being realistic enough? If so, perhaps it is but you haven't found the right way to go about it. There are several ways to achieve the same thing; you just have to be open to options. You may think that your mind doesn't work like that, in which case ask a friend, and of course I would also say ask God. Listen. Listen to what others are saying around you. It's surprising what you can pick up from other people's conversations. I once overheard a discussion between two women who were giving absolute opposite opinions on the same matter and it occurred to me that I had never considered it from the point of view of one of the women. Right, wrong or not sure – test the waters. What's the worst...

I grew up in a loving family setting, but my mother didn't encourage me and my two sisters to voice our own opinions. We just went along with whatever was said. Don't rock the boat. I was twelve when my father died and it was the most difficult time I can remember. Things seemed to be stable up until then, but without him there I was the youngest left at home with my mother. Both sisters were married and had left home. My mother was fifty six, a widow with one adolescent, stroppy daughter left in her care. It was an odd, strange, weird time. There was no manual to tell either of us how to behave. There still isn't! So we somehow managed to bungle along. It wasn't easy for either of us. My sisters helped where and when they could but they, too, were grieving our father.

It therefore came as a great revelation to me when I realised many years later that I could actually voice my opinion and it was ok. That I could have a row with someone and that, too, was ok because you don't end up hating someone because you have a difference of opinion. I currently attend a small group where two people often debate an issue from their own corner and I still find it interesting to listen and watch their responses. It's all ok because there is a mark of respect between them and they are both very eloquent and have a great command of the English language, but they each stand their ground and usually end up agreeing to disagree. It's ok to do that.

How many times have I reminded you in this book and myself that we are all different? We are. We are wonderfully made. Whatever our disabilities or attitude or looks, we are all made for a reason and put on this earth to make the best out of what we are given.

Some time ago I was teaching a group of adults and my stock phrase was, "We'll work with what we've got." That referred to the students as well as the resources. What have you been given? What would you like to change? Is it possible to change the situation or could you change your attitude about it or your perception of a person to make the difference? Work with what you've got. Be grateful about the small things and they will increase.

chapter nine

cancer – the facts

What do I know about the facts of cancer? Only that I have had it and seen others go through its gruelling trudge in an effort to become better. Some have survived, others haven't, but they've all had a go at beating it by one degree or another.

According to the World Health Organisation, 'More than 30% of cancer could be prevented, mainly by not using tobacco, having a healthy diet, being physically active and moderating the use of alcohol.' I didn't smoke, have been a vegetarian since I was twenty (over forty years), hardly ever drink alcohol and at the time of my diagnosis was playing badminton once a week and walking the dog twice a day. So how does that work?

We're all different and no one can predict who is going to get cancer and who is not. Of course, lifestyle will play a big part, but when I asked my consultant why it had attacked me and questioned if he was sure, were they definitely the correct medical notes and all the other questions that spring to mind in this situation, he just smiled. But, I continued, I am a vegetarian, don't drink or smoke etc., etc., but all he could answer is that, "We don't know yet. There's a lot more research to be done."

At the time this felt like an unsatisfactory response, but now I can see that it is true. The more research that is carried out, the more time we spend on trying to detect where cancer is going to strike next, I suppose the more we will know. It is only through more knowledge that we can find out how to live and eat and exercise well enough to avoid the risk. Furthermore, we need to be able to be one step ahead of it and use predictions wisely.

There are more than a hundred types of cancer and therefore over a hundred different systems in the body that have to be examined. How can we ever keep up with this? You have to believe that we will; that one day cancer, like other diseases that have been extinguished, will be no more. It has to be a possibility. A probability.

If you take a look at the Cancer Research website, you will find lots of information. Too much if you've just been diagnosed, in my opinion. But take what you find useful from it. There are pages on drugs, cancer myths, their research, fundraising and much more. Other sites include Breast Cancer Research, an international peer-reviewed online journal; Breast Cancer Now, who claim to be the UK's largest breast cancer charity dedicated to funding research into the disease; Breast Cancer Care, claiming to be the only UK-wide charity providing care, information and support to people affected by breast cancer; MacMillan Cancer Support, who state on their website that they are there to support and help people take back some control in their life, helping with money worries and advice about work or listening if you just want to talk; LYLAC, standing for Live your Life after Cancer, run by two life coaches and offering help for people to move forward after cancer; Wessex Cancer Trust, whose website will tell you that they exist to provide local support for people living with or are affected by cancer, irrespective of age, stage and the type of cancer. The websites are given at the end of this book and were accurate at the time of going to print.

These are all sources of information and assistance, and can be of comfort when you initially just want to know what is happening to your body. Of course, some individuals just won't want to delve into the depths of knowledge and are content to let the medics do what they will and endure the consequences. That's fine. We are all different.

Both the medical facts and the individual, emotional stories I have been told contributed to this book. During my research some women have relayed tales of unimaginable sorrow, of operations going wrong, of relationships changing, of secondary cancers and those that have spread. It has all been very sad, which will account for the ten-year delay in writing this book. We often put off things we want to do out of self-preservation – I didn't want to revisit that time. But – and the but is very big here – there have also been some amusing tales. The latter are facts, too, because without the addition of humour it can be extremely difficult to get through those tough times. The times when you question if you're going to make it. If you will see your children grow up. If your spouse is about to be bereaved. Difficult times raising lots of questions.

I am not arrogant enough to lead you along any of the paths that may be spread out before you now, but I feel strongly that everyone should be given the facts. Not just statistics about survival rate if you reject chemotherapy, not just the amount cancer drugs have improved, not about the consequences of your decision about your body and medical care, but hard, individual facts. And that's difficult for all concerned. You have to ask questions sometimes and not just accept the first answer that is given. I found myself referring to several different sources of information to reach the conclusion on how I wanted to move forward. In the very beginning, I suggested that I would opt to do nothing about the cancer. However, this is hardly ever a sensible option. But find out and go with what you are comfortable with.

Currently, there's a lot of support around and I've mentioned some of the organisations that are in operation at the time of going to print, but depending on where you live, there may be many more.

Friends and family may be a helpful source of support but some people don't know what to say and may stay away. It's hard for the onlooker. Most people want to help and for those who are struggling to find a way, it falls to you to give them time, space and understanding. I found some people's reactions to be quite blunt, but they were unsure how to express their views to me and that's how I received them. It has been said that giving and receiving comments is like passing the salt – it's only when you take it and use it that you know you have got the right thing.

chapter ten

a reflection

It seems ironic that as I near writing the end of a book on how we must stand up to cancer, how we must be strong and not let it win, that I receive a call from my sister that they have found another tumour in her body, this time in her kidney. This is bad news. Breast cancer three times and now another diagnosis on top of it all. A very testing time for her and for all of us who believe in a God who heals and protects us. However, her faith is strong and He has the power to heal and that's what keeps us going.

If my journey had been different, if I had stayed with my husband through it all, what would life be like now? If I hadn't got pregnant when I first did, how would our family tree sit now? We only have one chance in this life. So grab it with both hands. Some people believe in the afterlife – I believe in a Heaven where there is no suffering, no tears and no war. What if that could happen while we were still here on Earth? Can you imagine what it could be like? I can't, either. So we have to go through these trials and problems that are sent. We have to work with what we've got or else we just give up. In my book, that's not an option. We have to strive for more, for better.

When I started writing this book, I had just recovered from my operation and I was full of energy – well, relatively speaking – and I wanted to tell the world what it's like to have breast cancer and that it's not the end of the world. But for some people it is the end. I've come to realise that there are a great number of people going through what I've been through and they don't feel the need to write a book or tell the world that, actually, it's ok and you come through it. Why my journey should be any different and my response in any way better, worse, changed, altered or whatever word you want to insert there, I don't know. But I do know that I am grateful for the road I was led along – at times with no choice.

There are good things that come out of all situations; you just have to look for them. Sometimes you have to look harder than others when they are obviously staring you in the face. This book has been waiting on my virtual bookcase for over ten years. For some time I refused to acknowledge it needed writing at all and for the reasons I mentioned: why would anyone want to read my thoughts and feelings? Maybe some will resonate with you. It is, therefore, my hope that my words will encourage and motivate someone, somewhere out there. I am also aware that I may offend others and be rubbished by some. This is the risk any author takes and I will examine comments received and consider my script in their light. At this precise moment, before my manuscript even hits the printers (let alone gets past my publisher and copy editor) I know that what I have written is true to what I feel and reflects my own opinions.

Wherever you are right now, you have been blessed in one way or another. Even if you don't feel like it right now, you have. Do you have a home, a bed, food, a family or even a pet? If you can give one answer of 'yes' to any of these, believe me, you are blessed. There are always people worse off than you, just look around to the Developing World, to those who have lost their homes. And take a look at the alcoholic, the drug addict, the divorcee, the bereaved. Even they have something if they strive long enough to look for it, but chances are you are in a better place than any of these people.

A long time ago I worked in a drug and rehabilitation centre where I taught literacy and IT. The amazing poetry and stories that came out of that centre were incredibly cathartic for the residents and I encouraged them to write their own magazine. This happened and I could visibly see the authors (for that's what they were) stand tall and feel proud and confident of what they had achieved. We weren't allowed to sell the magazine but a suggested donation of a pound was given. As you can imagine, to someone in a rehab centre who has nothing, it was immensely empowering to them that people would pay for their work. We used the money to buy books for the internal library.

I often have to remind myself that I have been through many life traumas, maybe not as many as you, but enough to know that I can manage. My strength lies in God. Maybe that resonates with you, maybe not.

Women are brave and very strong. You can be too. Take hold of what you have right now and make it into what you want it to be. Our opportunities are limitless but we don't always see that when we are in the middle of a situation where we have to make a decision or make something more out of the little we have right now. Keep going, press on through and you will see the end. It is in sight, just look ahead. Look up.

Recently, I read a lovely saying which I want to pass on to you now: 'If you see someone without a smile, give them one of yours.' These days we may be concerned that people think we're just plain odd if we smile at them, but in my experience if you smile and walk on or smile and look away it can make their day. You may not even know it, but you could be the only person to give them a smile that day.

I am fortunate. I have been blessed and I know that I have a lot of people around me who are forgiving, and not only that, but have forgotten what I was like during my dark times. Like Jesus, He not only forgives our sins but He *forgets* them too. 'As far as the East is from the West, so far has he removed our transgressions (sins/mistakes) from us.' (Psalm 103) Believe it. You don't have to go through life carrying a heavy burden of knowing that you have done something wrong. It can be lifted from you and placed somewhere else. Taken away, removed, so that you can get on with your life as God has planned it for you.

I am also fortunate in that I have a husband who understands me. Rare, I know. We manage to work along together very well. Of course we have had our ups and downs – what worse 'down' can there be than separation? But through it all, we have been together longer than we haven't and that says something about a determination to make a relationship work. In these days when there are so many divorces and couples living together – what are we looking for? A perfect marriage? I don't believe there is such a thing. Both parties have to practise tolerance and keep a sense of humour. Not always easy to do, but possible. Very possible.

If stress is acknowledged as a contributory factor to getting cancer, then we need to watch our stress levels. How important is that job, promotion, goal or whatever you are chasing at the moment? How would it feel if you just were to let it go for a moment? Is it worth it? Ask yourself and answer yourself after you have given it some thought.

It can be the case that people don't fully understand, or aren't aware of the stress levels they are under until they stop. I was once told that no one is indispensable, but at the time I didn't believe it. Why can we not hear what others are trying to tell us for our own good? Maybe because we think that no one else can do the job we do as well as we do. *They* don't understand. However, it is sometimes that they just do it differently to how we used to carry out the tasks. Occasionally, this has to be recognised and maybe their actions have made the journey to the end result in an improved manner. Let's take the opportunities that are laid before us – and they are there on a daily basis – to praise others, give them a metaphorical pat on the back, help them to feel good about themselves. Certainly in a work situation you will get more out of your staff if you acted like this. Outside the office, we can learn to live in a more companionable way, giving praise and gratification when a situation arises and it is appropriate to do so.

How easy it is to get stuck in the 'we've always done it this way' scenario and so no one backs you when you see an easier/better/more efficient way to achieve the same end. Try just letting go and sometimes through your actions things can change. It's no good harbouring a grudge because you're not being listened to. Try grace! Graciously accept how things are being done and go along with it. If something is really, really important to you, try to get a few other people on your side, and if possible model how you can see it being done. Sometimes actions do speak louder than words. And sometimes we have to go it alone to prove this.

a poem to cancer

you took away my sister
you tried the same with me,
I don't want to make an enemy of you
but all I'm saying is please,
please just go away,
leave the human race in peace,
take your nasty little tumours
and run until you're done;
don't try to wipe us out
or try to make us weak.
The strong of us will stand,
research until we find
the antidote to finish you
and give us peace of mind.
Be in no doubt that day will come
and there will be no more pain,
suffering, sadness and death
because of the little 'c'.

Anon

references

www.who.int/features/factfiles/cancer/facts/en/index9.html
World Health Organisation fact files

www.wessexcancer.org.uk
Wessex Cancer Trust

www.cancerresearchuk.org
Cancer Research UK

www.breastcancernow.org
Breast Cancer Now

www.breastcancercare.org.uk
Breast Cancer Care

www.macmillan.org.uk
MacMillian Cancer Support

www.lylac.net
LYLAC

To contact the author email: smallc1@outlook.com

appendix

What is cancer?

Cancer can start in any place in the body. It starts when cells grow out of control and crowd out normal cells. This makes it hard for the body to function the way it should.

Why are cancer cells powerful?

All the cells in our bodies usually work together as a community. However, if a cell acquires a gene mutation that makes it multiply when it should not, or helps it survive when other cells die, it has an advantage over the others. Eventually, the abnormal cells acquire mutation in more genes, causing uncontrolled growth. These abnormal cells have a competitive advantage over normal cells. Think of natural selection in evolution, where a species that produces more offspring has a better chance of survival and this is how cancer cells survive and multiply.

What are tumours?

Most cancers form a lump called a tumour or a growth. But not all lumps are cancer. A piece of the lump is cut out and looked at to find out if it's cancer. Lumps that are not cancerous are called benign; lumps that are cancerous are called malignant.

There are some cancers, like leukaemia (cancer of the blood), that don't form tumours. They grow in the blood cells or other cells of the body.

What stage is the cancer?

The doctor also needs to know if and how far the cancer has spread from where it started. This is called the cancer stage. You may have heard other people say that their cancer was stage 1 or stage 2. Knowing the stage of the cancer helps the doctor decide what type of treatment is best.

For each type of cancer there are tests that can be done to figure out the stage of the cancer. As a rule, a lower stage (such as a stage 1 or 2) means that the cancer has not spread very much. A higher number (such as a stage 3 or 4) means it has spread more. Stage 4 is the highest stage.

How is cancer treated?

The most common treatments for cancer are surgery, chemotherapy and radiation.

Surgery can be used to take out the cancer. The surgeon might also take out some or all of the body part the cancer affects. For breast cancer, part (or all) of the breast might be removed. For prostate cancer, the prostate gland might be taken out. Surgery is not used for all types of cancer. For example, blood cancers like leukaemia are best treated with drugs.

Chemo (short for chemotherapy) is the use of drugs to kill cancer cells or slow their growth. Some chemo can be given by IV (into a vein through a needle) and others by a pill you swallow. Because chemo drugs travel to nearly all parts of the body, they are useful for cancer that has spread.

Radiation is also used to kill or slow the growth of cancer cells. It can be used alone or with surgery or chemo. Radiation treatment is like getting an x-ray, it doesn't hurt.

Why did this happen to me?

People with cancer often ask, "What did I do wrong?" or "Why me?" Doctors don't know for sure what causes cancer. When doctors can't give a cause, people may come up with their own ideas about why it happened.

Some people think they're being punished for something they did or didn't do in the past. Most people wonder if they did something to cause the cancer.

If you're having these feelings, you're not alone. Thoughts and beliefs like this are common for people with cancer. You need to know that cancer is not a punishment for your past actions. Try to not blame yourself or focus on looking for ways you might have prevented cancer. Cancer is not your fault, and there's almost never a way to find out what caused it. Instead, focus on taking good care of yourself now.

Thoughts on talking about cancer

It can be difficult to talk about cancer, even with the people you love. Discovering you have cancer can stir many feelings, such as sadness, anger and fear. Sometimes it's hard to know how you're feeling, much less talk to others about it.

Those close to you may also have a hard time talking about cancer. It's not easy for them to know what to say to help you or make you feel better. Allow them to help you if and when you need support and be clear about what you need and what you don't want.

Cancer words you may hear and their meaning:

Benign (be-NINE): a tumour that's not cancerous.

Biopsy (BY-op-see): taking out a piece of tissue to see if cancer cells are in it.

Cancer (CAN-sur): a word used to describe more than 100 diseases in which cells grow out of control; or a tumour with cancer in it.

Chemotherapy (key-mo-THER-uh-pee): the use of drugs to treat disease. The word most often refers to drugs used to treat cancer. Sometimes it's just called 'chemo'.

Malignant (muh-LIG-nunt): having cancer in it.

Metastasis/Metastasized   (meh-TAS-tuh-sis/meh-TAS-tuh-sized)**:** the spread of cancer cells to distant parts of the body through the lymph system or bloodstream.

Oncologist (on-KAHL-uh-jist)**:** a doctor who treats people who have cancer.

Radiotherapy (ray-dee-O-THER-uh-pee)**:** the use of high-energy rays, like x-rays, to treat cancer.

Remission (re-MISH-un): when signs or symptoms of cancer are all or partly gone.

Stage: a word that tells whether a cancer has spread, and if so, how far.

PRINTED AND BOUND BY:
Copytech (UK) Limited trading as Printondemand-worldwide,
9 Culley Court, Bakewell Road, Orton Southgate.
Peterborough, PE2 6XD, United Kingdom.

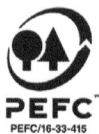